The Infection Preventionist's Guide to the Lab

Edited by

Patricia A. Kulich, RN, CIC
David L. Taylor, PhD, D(ABMM)

Printed in the United States of America
First edition, June 2012
Reprinted, January 2020
ISBN: 1-933013-52-4

All inquiries about *The Infection Preventionist's Guide to the Lab* or other APIC products and services may be addressed to:

APIC

1275 K Street NW, Suite 1000
Washington, DC 20005-4006
Phone: 202-789-1890
Fax: 202-789-1899
Email: products@apic.org
Web: www.apic.org

Table of Contents

Foreword

Diagnostics, surveillance, and disease trend analysis are increasingly critical parts of a comprehensive infection prevention program. For this reason, infection preventionists and laboratory professionals need to understand the roles each must play and work together to improve patient outcomes. To facilitate this, APIC partnered with the American Society for Microbiology (ASM) to create the IP Col-Lab-oration project, part of the Building Bridges program.*

The goals of the IP Col-lab-oration project are as follows:

- To increase communication and understanding between laboratory professionals and infection preventionists
- To educate in the common areas of infection prevention and microbiology that include surveillance via diagnostics/ screening for resistant organism carriage, and targeted disease trending over time.
- To equip infection preventionists and laboratory professionals with educational resources and tools that will lead to improved outcomes through better integration of effort and communication.

The Infection Preventionist's Guide to the Lab was developed to provide infection preventionists with a basic understanding of various lab tests and microbiology disciplines. This book supports infection preventionists in making informed decisions about surveillance and patient placement. While the development of this book began before the launch of the IP Col-lab-oration Project, it became clear that the goals of the book and the project were aligned. As a result, our collaborative partner, ASM, provided additional technical review of this resource.

APIC is grateful to the editors, David Taylor and Pat Kulich, the eleven chapter authors, additional contributors, and many reviewers from APIC and ASM who worked together to make this resource a reality.

Our hope is that this resource in conjunction with the IP Col-lab-oration Project will usher in a new era of improved infection prevention practice that lowers healthcare associated infection, reduces the trend of increasing antibiotic resistance in bacterial pathogens, and improves the quality of care given to all our patients. Those of us involved in this project are grateful for the opportunity to participate and share the excitement of our two great societies in the exciting future we will better share together.

Lillian A. Burns, MT, MPH, CIC and Lance R. Peterson, MD
Lead Clinical Advisors, IP Col-lab-oration project

** About Building Bridges: In the beginning of 2010, APIC created the Building Bridges program to improve patient outcomes by building bridges between infection preventionists and stakeholders across the continuum of care. Funded by educational grants, each project focuses on one specific area related to infection prevention and dives deep with a key society partner or partners. Guiding the project is a clinical advisory council of subject matter experts from each participating society. The advisory council produces educational programs and resources. To learn more about the Building Bridges program, visit www.apic.org/buildingbridges.*

Preface

This resource was created to help the infection preventionist better understand the laboratory and its applications to infection prevention. It covers many topics within the discipline of microbiology as well as the various functions of the laboratory itself. The authors were chosen due to their expertise in the laboratory field as well as their experience in or relationship to infection prevention.

This book is intended to be a quick reference guide rather than an exhaustive laboratory text. Each chapter focuses on a specific type of laboratory test or microbiology discipline and its applicability to the infection preventionist, and includes an introduction, one or more tables, and a list of references.

A collaborative relationship between infection prevention and the laboratory is important to achieve the common goal of improving patient outcomes. If readers have questions or need further clarification regarding a specific laboratory test or results, they are encouraged to consult with the clinical laboratory associated with their facility.

As editors, we are extremely proud of the hard work of all the contributing authors and content reviewers. We feel it will provide valuable insight into the world of the clinical laboratory and how that world impacts the practicing infection preventionist.

Good reading – and enjoy.

David Taylor, PhD, D(ABMM) and Pat Kulich, RN, CIC
Editors

Acknowledgments

The Association for Professionals in Infection Control and Epidemiology (APIC) acknowledges the valuable contributions of the following individuals:

Editors

Patricia A. Kulich, RN, CIC
Infection Preventionist (retired)
Grove City, OH

David L. Taylor, PhD, D(ABMM)
Infection Preventionist (retired)
Enon, OH

Authors

Kathy Aureden, MS, MT(ASCP)SI, CIC
Epidemiology Coordinator
Sherman Hospital
Elgin, IL

Clemence Cherson, MPA, CIC, CLS (ASCP)
Director, Infection Prevention and Control
St. Joseph Hospital
Bethpage, NY

Nancy E. Christy, MT, MSHA, CIC
Infection Preventionist
Georgetown University Hospital
Washington, DC

Jeanne Dickman, MT(ASCP), CIC
Infection Preventionist
Department of Clinical Epidemiology
Wexner Medical Center at The Ohio State University and James Cancer Center
Columbus, OH

Lynn Slonim Fine, PhD, MPH, CIC
Infection Preventionist
Strong Memorial Hospital
Rochester, NY

Carolyn Fiutem, MT(ASCP), CIC
Infection Prevention Officer
TriHealth – Good Samaritan Hospital – Bethesda North Hospital
Cincinnati, OH

Geraldine S. Hall, PhD
Medical Director, Clinical Microbiology
Cleveland Clinic Foundation
Cleveland, OH

Lul Raka, MD, PhD
Faculty of Medicine
University of Prishtina and National Institute of Public Health of Kosova
Prishtina, Kosova

Justin Smyer, MLS(ASCP)CM, MPH
Infection Control Practitioner
Department of Clinical Epidemiology
Wexner Medical Center East at The Ohio State University
Columbus, OH

Carol Sykora, MT(ASCP), MEd, CIC
Infection Prevention Consultant
BJC Infection Prevention and Epidemiology Consortium - IPEC
St. Louis, MO

Contributors

Ana Budimir, MD,PhD
Clinical Hospital Centre Zagreb
Zagreb, Croatia

Smilja Kalenić, MD, PhD
Clinical Hospital Centre Zagreb
Zagreb, Croatia

Jill Midgett, MT, SM(ASCP)
Manager, Microbiology Laboratory
Lawrence and Memorial Hospital
New London, CT

Sallie Jo Rivera, RN, MSN, CIC
Infection Preventionist
Central Dupage Hospital
Winfield, IL

Susan Wagoner, BS, MT(ASCP)SM
Lead Microbiologist
Sherman Hospital
Elgin, IL

Dick Zoutman, MD, FRCPC
Faculty of Health Sciences, Queen's University at Kingston
Chief of Staff, Quinte Health Care
Belleville, Ontario, Canada

Reviewers: Association for Professionals in Infection Control and Epidemiology

Lillian A. Burns, MT, MPH, CIC
Administrative Director of Infection Control/ Epidemiology
Staten Island University Hospital
Staten Island, NY

Carol Elder, BS, CIC
Infection Control Specialist
Mt. Carmel West
Columbus, OH

Candace Friedman, MPH, CIC
Director, Infection Control and Epidemiology
University of Michigan Hospitals and Health Centers
Ann Arbor, MI

Karen Swecker, RN, CIC
Infection Control Specialist
Mt. Carmel St. Ann's
Westerville, OH

Reviewers: American Society for Microbiology

Eileen M. Burd, PhD, D(ABMM)
Director, Clinical Microbiology Emory University Hospital
Associate Professor, Emory University School of Medicine
Department of Pathology 7 Laboratory Medicine and
Department of Medicine, Division of Infectious Diseases
Atlanta, GA

Patricia Charache, PhD
Program Director, Quality Assurance and Outcomes Research
Johns Hopkins Medical Institutions
Department of Pathology
Baltimore, MD

Chris Doern, PhD
Assistant Professor of Pathology
University of Texas Southwestern Department of Pathology
Children's Medical Center
Dallas, TX

Robert Fader, PhD
Section Chief, Microbiology/Virology Laboratories
Scott & White Healthcare
Temple, TX

Lance R. Petersen, MD
Epidemiologist
NorthShore University Health System
Evanston, IL

Yvette S. McCarter, PhD, D(ABMM)
Director, Clinical Microbiology Laboratory
University of Florida
Department of Pathology
Jacksonville, FL

Michael A. Pentella, PhD, D(ABMM)
Clinical Associate Professor
The University of Iowa, College of Public Health
Department of Epidemiology
University Hygienic Laboratory
Iowa City, IA

Paula Revell, PhD, D(ABMM)
Assist Professor of Pathology, Baylor College of Medicine
Director of Microbiology, Virology, Molecular Diagnostic Labs
Texas Children's Hospital
Houston, TX

Barbara E. Robinson-Dunn, PhD
Technical Director, Microbiology
William Beaumont Hospital
Clinical Pathology
Royal Oak, MI

Susan Sharp, PhD, D(ABMM), F(AAM)
Regional Director of Microbiology
Kaiser Permanente - NW
Portland, OR

Production Team

Anna Conger
Project Management
Editorial Oversight

Christina James
Project Support

Walter Josephs
Project Liaison – The IP Col-lab-oration Project

Meredith McClay
Maryland Comp
Book Design and Layout

Sarah Vickers
Cover Design

Chapter 1

Specimen Collection and Transport

Lul Raka, MD, PhD

Additional Contributors:
Dick Zoutman, MD, FRCPC
Smilja Kalenić, MD, PhD
Ana Budimir, MD, PhD

The diagnostic microbiology laboratory (DML) plays a pivotal role in patient care by providing information on a variety of microorganisms with clinical significance such as bacteria, fungi, viruses, and parasites. The primary goals of the DML are to identify the presence of pathogenic microorganisms in clinical samples, predict response to antimicrobial therapy, and assist the infection prevention department as needed in epidemiological investigation.

A variety of methods can be used to identify microorganisms in clinical specimens. Methods used in the DML in the diagnosis of infection are (1) classical methods (direct smear, culture, antigen detection, serological tests) and (2) molecular methods (hybridization, nucleic acid amplification, real-time amplification).

The DML is an essential component of an effective infection prevention program. Changes in microbiological diagnostic techniques, such as rapid diagnosis and typing methods, have strengthened the role of microbiology laboratory in infection prevention. The partnership between the infection preventionist and the DML medical microbiologist is crucial in combating healthcare-associated infections (HAIs).

The appropriate selection, collection, and transport of specimens to the DML is an essential part in the accurate laboratory identification of microorganisms that cause infections which affect patient care and infection prevention.

Specimen collection guidelines include:

- Use standard precautions for collecting and handling all clinical specimens.
- Utilize appropriate collection device(s).
- Use sterile equipment and aseptic technique to collect specimens.
- Collect specimens during the acute phase of illness (or within 2 to 3 days for viral infections).
- Collect specimens before administration of antibiotics wherever possible.
- Avoid contamination with indigenous flora from surrounding tissues, organs, or secretions.
- Optimize the capture of anaerobic bacteria from specimens by using proper procedures.
- Collect a sufficient volume of specimen to ensure that all tests requested may be performed. Inadequate amounts of specimen may yield false-negative results.
- Label specimens properly with patient's name and identification number, source, specific site, date, time of collection, and initials of collector.
- Provide clear and specific instructions on proper collection techniques to patients when they must collect their own specimens.

Transportation guidelines include:

- All specimens must be promptly transported to the laboratory, preferably within 2 hours of collection.
  - Delays or exposure to temperature extremes compromises the test results.
- Specimens should be transported in a container designed to ensure survival of suspected agents.
  - Never refrigerate spinal fluid, genital, eye, or internal ear specimens because these samples may contain microorganisms sensitive to temperature extremes.
- Materials for transport must be labeled properly, packaged, and protected during transport.
  - A transport medium can be used to preserve the viability of microorganisms in clinical samples (e.g. Stuart, Amies, and Carey-Blair transport media).
- Use leak-proof specimen containers and transport them in sealable, leak-proof plastic bags.
- Never transport syringes with needles attached to the laboratory.
- Laboratories must have enforceable criteria for rejection of unsuitable specimens.

See Chapter 2 for additional information.

Table 1-1: Specimen Selection, Collection, and Transport by Body Site

Upper Respiratory Tract										
General Category	Laboratory Test	Indications	Specific Microbes	Specimen	Frequency	Test Type	Interpretation	Advantages/Disadvantages	Sample Transport	Key Points
Oral cavity	• Gram stain principally • Infrequently cultures	Oral lesions, suspicion of oral yeast infection ("thrush"), necrotizing gingivitis	*Candida* sp., *Fusobacterium* sp. or other anaerobes or spirochetes in cases of necrotizing gingivitis	• Swab of lesions or purulent material • Bacterial transport media	Once	Swab	• Gram stain reveals yeast • Gram stain reveals fusiform bacilli or spirochetes	Swabs not very sensitive or specific	Swab and transport within 2 hours to laboratory (≤2 h) at room temperature (RT)	Culture rarely indicated
Nares	Culture or polymerase chain reaction (PCR) for methicillin-resistant *Staphylococcus aureus* (MRSA)	Epidemiological screening for MRSA	MRSA	• Swab of anterior nares • Bacterial transport media	• Once at assessment • Repeat as needed clinically	Nasal swab	Positive culture or PCR indicates colonization with MRSA	• PCR very sensitive and specific but more costly • Specialized test	Swab and transport ≤2 h at RT	Concurrent cultures of wounds or perianal skin also recommended to compensate for lower sensitivity of nares culture method
Nasopharyngeal	• Viral cell culture, fluorescent antibody stain, rapid membrane antigen detection, or PCR • Bacterial culture	Viral testing (e.g., influenza), bacterial culture of certain pathogens	Influenza, parainfluenza, respiratory syncytial virus (RSV), other respiratory viruses, *Neisseria meningitidis*, *Bordetella pertussis*, *Corynebacterium diphtheriae*, *Streptococcus pneumoniae*, *Staphylococcus aureus*, *Hemophilus influenzae*, *Moraxella catarrhalis*, *Pseudomonas* species, oral anaerobes, occasionally fungi or other pathogens	• Swab placed into viral transport media • Swab placed into bacterial transport media	Once	Nasopharyngeal swab or aspirate	Detection of viral pathogens has high specificity but sensitivity highly variable depending on methods used	PCR for respiratory viruses is very sensitive and rapid if available	Swab and transport ≤2 h at RT	May cause coughing, requiring appropriate personal protective equipment (PPE) for person collecting the specimen

Table 1-1: Specimen Selection, Collection, and Transport by Body Site (*continued*)

Upper Respiratory Tract										
General Category	Laboratory Test	Indications	Specific Microbes	Specimen	Frequency	Test Type	Interpretation	Advantages/ Disadvantages	Sample Transport	Key Points
Sinuses	• Bacterial culture • Gram stain	Healthcare-associated sinusitis in a critical care setting, especially if on mechanical ventilation	*S. pneumoniae, S. aureus, H. influenzae, M. catarrhalis, Pseudomonas* species, oral anaerobes, occasionally fungi or other pathogens such as coliforms	• Specimen placed into sterile collection device and delivered to laboratory immediately • Swab of nasal mucus NOT an acceptable specimen	Once and possibly repeated if clinically required	Direct maxillary puncture by surgeon or aspiration of sinus cavity under direct visualization	Predominant growth of a pathogen that is also seen in the Gram stain suggests pathogenic role	Aspiration of the maxillary sinus by puncture or direct visualization requires specialist to perform	Swab and transport ≤2 h at RT	
Throat	• Tests for MRSA as described for nares • Culture for *C. diphtheriae* • Culture or PCR for *B. pertussis*	Screening for MRSA, diphtheria, or pertussis	MRSA, *C. diphtheria, B. pertussis*	Swab placed into bacterial transport media	• Once at assessment • Repeat as needed clinically	Swab of posterior pharyngeal wall and tonsils including exudates or purulent material	• For MRSA, as for nares • *C. diphtheriae* requires toxigenic testing to determine its disease-producing potential	• "Cough plates" no longer recommended for pertussis • If clinical suspicion high for diphtheria or pertussis then appropriate infection prevention and notification of public health authorities required at the time of specimen collection	Swab and transport ≤2 h at RT	• Always speak with microbiology laboratory if diphtheria or pertussis considered because special handling is required • Throat swab contraindicated for patients with suspected epiglottitis

Table 1-1: Specimen Selection, Collection, and Transport by Body Site *(continued)*

Lower Respiratory Tract										
General Category	Laboratory Test	Indications	Specific Microbes	Specimen	Frequency	Test Type	Interpretation	Advantages/ Disadvantages	Sample Transport	Key Points
Expectorated sputum	Bacterial, fungal cultures	Healthcare-associated pneumonia or tracheobronchitis	*S. pneumoniae, H. influenzae, B. catarrhalis,* coliforms, *S. aureus, Pseudomonas* species, other glucose nonfermenters, *Legionella* species, mycobacteria species	Sputum, aspirates from endotracheal tube or tracheostomy	• As clinically indicated but not normally more often than once per week • Not for surveillance purposes, only as directed by clinical symptoms or radiological changes	Expectorated, aspirated specimen	• Very challenging to interpret for bacterial infections • Isolation of bacteria or aspergillus does not in itself indicate the presence of lower respiratory tract infection • Clinical or epidemiological criteria for pneumonia require other features such as increased oxygen requirements, radiological changes, etc. • *Legionella* species not expected to be a contaminant and considered a significant finding	• Due to difficulties in interpretation of sputum samples, consideration should be given to broncho-alveolar lavage (BAL) or protected bronchoscopic brush specimens using quantitative microbiological methods for diagnosis of healthcare-associated pneumonia. • Urine antigen for *Legionella pneumophila* • PCR for *L. pneumophila*	Sterile container, transport ≤2 h at RT	Legionella specimens should not be collected in saline; sterile water is best
Induced sputum	Viral detection	Healthcare-associated viral respiratory infection	Respiratory viruses such as influenza, RSV	Induced sputum collected in sterile bottle					Sterile container, transport ≤2 h at RT	

Table 1-1: Specimen Selection, Collection, and Transport by Body Site *(continued)*

Lower Respiratory Tract										
General Category	Laboratory Test	Indications	Specific Microbes	Specimen	Frequency	Test Type	Interpretation	Advantages/ Disadvantages	Sample Transport	Key Points
• Broncho-alveolar lavage (BAL), endotracheal aspirate • Bronchial brushing	• Bacterial, fungal cultures; direct fluorescent stain or PCR for *Pneumocystis jiroveci* • Viral detection	Healthcare-associated pneumonia or tracheobronchitis, healthcare-associated viral respiratory infection where sputum is not specific enough	As above; better for *P. jiroveci* than sputum specimens	• Bronchoscopically obtained lavage of a lung segment where bronchoscope is wedged into a segmental bronchus and lung segment is flushed with up to 100 mL of sterile saline that is aspirated back through the bronchoscope • Alternative is protected bronchial brush that is placed into affected lung area through bronchoscope	• As clinically indicated but not normally more often than once per week • Not for surveillance purposes • Only as directed by clinical symptoms or radiological changes	• Bronchoscopically collected BAL collected in a sterile bottle, or protected specimen brush collected 1.0 mL of sterile saline • Use sterile water for *Legionella* species	• Specimens are cultured using a quantitative method to differentiate pathogens from contaminants • Exact cut-off values depend on individual laboratory procedures • *P. jiroveci* fluorescent antibody stain or PCR very sensitive and specific	These specialized specimens require a bronchoscopy to be performed, which is not always possible in patients with severe respiratory failure	Sterile container, transport ≤2 h at RT	• In general, where a significant lower respiratory tract infection is considered, BAL is the preferred specimen if it can be safely collected • Immediate transportation to the microbiology laboratory is necessary • Due to the risks of bronchoscopy in critically ill patients, advanced planning with the medical microbiologist is highly recommended

Table 1-1: Specimen Selection, Collection, and Transport by Body Site *(continued)*

Blood and Intravascular Devices

General Category	Laboratory Test	Indications	Specific Microbes	Specimen	Frequency	Test Type	Interpretation	Advantages/ Disadvantages	Sample Transport	Key Points
Blood cultures	Aerobic and anaerobic culture of blood for bacteria and yeast	Clinical suspicion of bacteremia or septic shock	Many: *S. aureus, S. pneumoniae,* meningococci, enterococci, coliforms, *Pseudomonas* species, nonfermenting Gram-negative bacilli (*Acinetobacter, Stenotrophomonas maltophilia, Burkholderia, Moraxella*), yeasts	• Blood from properly cleaned and disinfected vein site • Less desirable from central venous catheter due to increased risk of contamination of the specimen • On average, 30–40 mL of blood per septic episode in adults taken before administration of antimicrobials if at all possible • Volume in children based on body weight	• One venipuncture drawing 20 mL of blood divided evenly between an aerobic and anaerobic bottle (i.e., 10 mL per bottle constituting one set of blood cultures) • Repeat at new venipuncture site • If endovascular infection considered, then draw a third set 1 or more hours after first two sets taken	• Whole blood aseptically drawn into blood culture bottle • Normally place 10 mL into each bottle for adults and larger children, and take no less than two sets (four bottles) per septic episode to ensure >95% sensitivity • Blood cultures incubated in most semi-automated detection systems for 5 days	• Typical pathogens such as *S. aureus* always considered significant • Typical skin flora such as coagulase-negative staphylococcus species, *Corynebacterium* species, etc., identified in only one set of bottles is highly suggestive of a contaminant	• Single sets of blood cultures of limited value with reduced sensitivity to detect a bacteremia and are to be avoided • Available blood culture systems not generally able to detect filamentous fungi; in such cases, lysis centrifugation tubes may be needed or alternative methods (e.g., serology)	Blood culture bottles, transport ≤2 h at RT	• Proper skin preparation with 70% alcohol and chlorhexidine will reduce the risk of contamination to less than 2% of specimens • Follow specified protocol of your microbiology laboratory
Central venous catheter	• Aerobic culture for bacteria and yeast • Semi-quantitative roll plate or sonication (detects intra-luminal infection) methods	Clinical suspicion of central venous catheter–related bacteremia	Many: *S. aureus, S. pneumoniae,* meningococci, enterococci, coliforms, *Pseudomonas* species, nonfermenting Gram-negative bacilli (*Acinetobacter, Stenotrophomonas maltophilia, Burkholderia, Moraxella*), yeasts	• Aseptically cut off terminal 5 cm of the catheter and place in sterile tube or bottle • Transport immediately to microbiology laboratory • Take concurrent blood cultures at the same time as described previously	• Only if there is a suspicion of central venous catheter causing a bacteremia • Do not routinely send venous catheter tips for culture if there is no suspicion of catheter-related bacteremia	• Catheter tip is rolled on bacterial agar • Concurrent blood cultures incubated as described	If >15 colonies cultured, considered significant if concurrent blood cultures also positive for the same pathogen	Careful attention to aseptic technique in cutting off the catheter segment required	Sterile screw-cap tube or cup, container, ≤15 min at RT	Catheter tips should be sent to the microbiology laboratory only with concurrent blood cultures to establish the presence of a bacteremia

Table 1-1: Specimen Selection, Collection, and Transport by Body Site (*continued*)

Sterile Body Sites and Fluids										
General Category	Laboratory Test	Indications	Specific Microbes	Specimen	Frequency	Test Type	Interpretation	Advantages/ Disadvantages	Sample Transport	Key Points
Abdominal abscess, biliary fluid	• Aerobic and anaerobic bacterial culture • Yeast culture	Suspicion of intra-abdominal, pelvic, or hepatic abscesses	*S. aureus,* enterococci, coliforms, *Pseudomonas* species, *Bacteroides* species, *Clostridium* species, other anaerobes, and *Candida* species or other yeasts	• Aseptically collected abscess fluid at time of surgery or by direct percutaneous aspiration • Specimen should be placed into anaerobic collection tube for optimal recovery of all pathogens	Once at time of surgery or by direct percutaneous aspiration	Aerobic and anaerobic bacterial cultures on multiple media to identify all potential pathogens	• Correlation with Gram stain and culture results essential • Classical pathogens easy to interpret • When patient has been on prolonged antibiotic therapy, coagulase negative staphylococcus species, enterococci, and yeasts may be the only pathogens discovered	• Early acquisition of the specimen in the course of the infection is ideal • Results more difficult to interpret in face of prior antibiotic therapy	• Anaerobic transport system, sterile tube or blood culture bottle ≤15 min at RT • Rapid delivery to laboratory is essential	• Do not take specimen from preexisting drainage collection device as this has an unacceptable risk of significant contamination • Swabs not adequate, collect liquid specimen
Ascites	• Aerobic and anaerobic bacterial culture • Yeast culture • Cell count and differential count of fluid	Suspicion of primary (spontaneous) or secondary peritonitis	• *S. aureus,* enterococci, coliforms, *Pseudomonas* species, *Bacteroides* species, *Clostridium* species, other anaerobes, and *Candida* species or other yeasts • Spontaneous bacterial peritonitis can also be caused by *S. pneumoniae*	• Aseptically aspirate ascites fluid • Place into anaerobic collection tube or sterile bottle • Additional 10 mL should be placed into aerobic blood culture bottle to increase yield of bacterial pathogens • Cell count in appropriate container for hematology laboratory	• Once at time of suspicion of peritonitis • May be repeated during therapy if there is no response to treatment	• Aerobic and anaerobic bacterial cultures on multiple media to identify all potential pathogens • Cell count and differential count on fluid	• >250 polymorphonuclear neutrophils (PMN) per mL compatible with spontaneous bacterial peritonitis, higher counts seen in secondary bacterial peritonitis • Elevated PMNs with positive cultures prove diagnosis of peritonitis	• Placing some but not all of the ascites fluid in a blood culture bottle at the patient's bedside improved yield of the cultures • It is still important to send fluid in sterile containers for Gram stain, cell counts, and bacterial culture onto agar media as well	• Anaerobic transport system, sterile tube or blood culture bottle ≤15 min at RT • Rapid delivery to laboratory is essential	Other forms of peritonitis to consider are culture negative neutrophilic ascites and monomicrobial nonneutrophilic bacterial ascites

Table 1-1: Specimen Selection, Collection, and Transport by Body Site *(continued)*

Sterile Body Sites and Fluids

General Category	Laboratory Test	Indications	Specific Microbes	Specimen	Frequency	Test Type	Interpretation	Advantages/ Disadvantages	Sample Transport	Key Points
Peritoneal dialysis fluid	• Aerobic and anaerobic bacterial culture • Yeast culture • Cell count and differential count of fluid	Suspicion of peritoneal dialysis catheter-related peritonitis	• *Staphylococcus epidermidis*, *S. aureus*, *Candida* species, *Pseudomonas aeruginosa*, or *S. maltophilia* • Rare cases of mycobacterial infection	• Aseptically collected peritoneal dialysis fluid through the catheter into anaerobic collection tube or sterile bottle • Additional 10 mL should be placed into aerobic blood culture bottles to increase yield of bacterial pathogens • Cell count in appropriate container for hematology laboratory	• Once at time of clinical suspicion of peritoneal dialysis catheter-related peritonitis • May be repeated during therapy if response incomplete (see above)	• Aerobic and anaerobic bacterial cultures on multiple media to identify all potential pathogens • Cell count and differential count on fluid	• >250 polymorphonuclear neutrophils (PMN) per mL compatible with spontaneous bacterial peritonitis, higher counts seen in secondary bacterial peritonitis • Elevated PMNs with positive cultures prove diagnosis of peritonitis	• Placing some but not all of the ascites fluid in a blood culture bottle at the patient's bedside improved yield of the cultures • It is still important to send fluid in sterile containers for Gram stain, cell counts, and bacterial culture onto agar media as well	• Anaerobic transport system, sterile tube or blood culture bottle ≤15 min at RT • Rapid delivery to laboratory is essential	Culture of the peritoneal dialysis catheter tip is not appropriate
Amniotic fluid	• Aerobic and anaerobic bacterial culture • Yeast culture	Suspicion of intraabdominal, pelvic, or hepatic abscesses	*S. aureus*, enterococci, coliforms, *Pseudomonas* species, *Bacteroides* species, *Clostridium* species, other anaerobes, and *Candida* species or other yeasts	• Aseptically collected abscess fluid at time of surgery or by direct percutaneous aspiration • Specimen should be placed into anaerobic collection tube for optimal recovery of all pathogens	Once at time of surgery or by direct percutaneous aspiration	Aerobic and anaerobic bacterial cultures on multiple media to identify all potential pathogens	• Correlation with Gram stain and culture results essential • Classical pathogens easy to interpret • When patient has been on prolonged antibiotic therapy, coagulase negative staphylococcus species, enterococci, and yeasts may be the only pathogens discovereds	• Fluid collected through a vaginal swab not acceptable specimen due to contamination with vaginal flora • Collect by percutaneous aspiration, at surgery, or by aseptically placed intrauterine catheter	• Anaerobic transport system, sterile tube or blood culture bottle ≤15 min at RT • Rapid delivery to laboratory is essential	Swabs of placenta not an appropriate specimen due to contamination by vaginal flora

Table 1-1: Specimen Selection, Collection, and Transport by Body Site (*continued*)

Sterile Body Sites and Fluids										
General Category	Laboratory Test	Indications	Specific Microbes	Specimen	Frequency	Test Type	Interpretation	Advantages/ Disadvantages	Sample Transport	Key Points
Synovial fluid	• Aerobic and anaerobic bacterial culture • Yeast culture • Cell count and differential count of fluid • Phase contrast microscopy for crystals	Clinical suspicion of septic arthritis of joint	*S. aureus, S. epidermidis,* enterococcus species, coliforms, *Pseudomonas* species, rarely yeast, fungi, mycobacteria, or nocardia	• Aseptic aspiration of joint or surgical exploration by arthrotomy with collection of joint fluid in anaerobic collection tube and into sterile bottle appropriate for cell count and microscopy for crystals • Collection should be before initiation of antimicrobial therapy if at all possible	Initially and repeated at time of second joint therapeutic lavage	• Aerobic and anaerobic bacterial cultures on multiple media to identify all potential pathogens • Cell count and differential count on fluid	For prosthetic joint infections very desirable to have specimens obtained at time of surgery as this facilitates interpretation of *S. epidermidis* and other low virulence pathogens	• Cultures by swabbing a chronic draining sinus lack sensitivity for the true pathogen in the joint space • Important to have proper aseptic aspiration or surgical samples	• Anaerobic transport system, sterile tube or blood culture bottle ≤15 min at RT • Rapid delivery to laboratory is essential	• Cell count and differential count as well as microscopy for crystals important
Pericardial fluid	• Aerobic and anaerobic bacterial culture • Yeast culture • Viral detection • Cell count and differential count of fluid	Clinical suspicion of pericarditis	*S. aureus, S. pneumoniae, H. influenzae, Pseudomonas* species, anaerobic bacteria, enterovirus, influenza, *Candida* species, *Histoplasmosis capsulatum, Aspergillus* species, mycobacteria	Aseptic aspiration of pericardial space or surgical exploration by pericardiotomy with collection of pericardial fluid in anaerobic collection tube, aerobic transport media, viral transport media, and into sterile bottle appropriate for cell count	• Once at time of clinical suspicion of pericarditis • May be repeated during therapy if response is incomplete; see above	• Aerobic and anaerobic bacterial, fungal, and mycobacterial cultures on multiple media to identify all potential pathogens • Viral culture and/or PCR • Cell count and differential count on fluid	• Any growth of a pathogen of significance • Most healthcare-associated-cases occur after cardiac surgery due to *S. aureus;* may be associated with sternal osteomyelitis	Some cases require pericardial window to drain the fluid	• Anaerobic transport system, sterile tube or blood culture bottle ≤15 min at RT • Rapid delivery to laboratory is essential	• Although uncommon, tuberculosis is still an important cause of pericarditis • Many cases undiagnosed due to viral etiology

Table 1-1: Specimen Selection, Collection, and Transport by Body Site *(continued)*

Sterile Body Sites and Fluids										
General Category	Laboratory Test	Indications	Specific Microbes	Specimen	Frequency	Test Type	Interpretation	Advantages/ Disadvantages	Sample Transport	Key Points
Pleural fluid	• Aerobic and anaerobic bacterial culture • Yeast culture • Mycobacterial and fungal cultures • Cell count and differential count of fluid • Lactate dehydrogenase (LDH), protein, pH to biochemistry laboratory also	Suspicion of pleural space infection, empyema, or tuberculosis	*S. pneumoniae, S. aureus, H. influenzae, Pseudomonas* species, anaerobic bacteria, oral aerobic bacteria, tuberculosis	• Aseptically collected pleural fluid at time of surgery or by direct percutaneous aspiration • Specimen should be placed into anaerobic collection tube for optimal recovery of all pathogens • Rapid delivery to microbiology laboratory essential	Initially and repeated during therapy if response is incomplete	• Aerobic and anaerobic bacterial, fungal, and mycobacterial cultures on multiple media to identify all potential pathogens • Cell count and differential count, LDH, protein, pH on fluid	• Accurate diagnosis with biochemical characteristics with elevated LDH, protein, and pH <7.0 essential as is culture • Biochemical characteristics and positive cultures of a pathogen confirms the diagnosis of empyema	Empyema occurs in 1%–2% of pneumonias and is therefore uncommon	• Anaerobic transport system, sterile tube or blood culture bottle ≤15 min at RT • Rapid delivery to laboratory is essential	Empyemas require tube drainage or surgical drainage/ decortication

Eye										
General Category	Laboratory Test	Indications	Specific Microbes	Specimen	Frequency	Test Type	Interpretation	Advantages/ Disadvantages	Sample Transport	Key Points
Conjunctiva	Conjunctival scraping for bacterial cultures, viral culture, fluorescent stain or PCR, chlamydia fluorescent stain or culture	Suspicion of conjunctivitis with purulent secretions	*H. influenzae, Neisseria gonorrhoeae, Chlamydia trachomatis, S. aureus,* herpes simplex virus (HSV), adenovirus	• Scrapings of conjunctiva or swabs of purulent material • Submit in bacterial, viral, and chlamydia transport media	Once and possibly repeated if clinically required	• Bacterial cultures • Viral cultures • Fluorescent antibody stain or PCR • Chlamydia fluorescent stain or culture	Positive results for a pathogen indicate a significant finding		Direct culture inoculation or swab transport ≤2 h	• Acute hemorrhagic conjunctivitis can occur in epidemics due to picornavirus • Epidemic keratoconjunctivitis due to adenovirus also occurs and is severe

Table 1-1: Specimen Selection, Collection, and Transport by Body Site *(continued)*

Eye										
General Category	Laboratory Test	Indications	Specific Microbes	Specimen	Frequency	Test Type	Interpretation	Advantages/ Disadvantages	Sample Transport	Key Points
Cornea	Corneal scraping for bacterial cultures, viral culture, fluorescent stain or PCR, *Acanthamoeba* fluorescent stain	Suspicion of corneal infection (keratitis) with pain, photophobia, increased secretions, and red eye	• *S. pneumoniae*, *S. aureus*, *P. aeruginosa*, *H. influenzae*, *M. catarrhalis*, HSV, varicella zoster virus • *Acanthamoeba* species (a protozoan)	• Corneal scrapings by qualified ophthalmologist with anesthesia • Multiple specimens recommended • Submit in bacterial transport media, viral transport media, and as freshly prepared smear onto glass slides for immediate staining with Giemsa stain and calcofluor white and viewed with fluorescent microscope	Once and possibly repeated if clinically required	• Bacterial cultures • Viral cultures • Fluorescent antibody stain or PCR • Giemsa stain and calcofluor fluorescent stain on scrapings	• Positive results for a pathogen indicate a significant finding • Positive Gram stain in 75% of bacterial cases • If diagnosis still not made, ophthalmologist may consider keratoplasty for diagnosis and treatment	*Acanthamoeba* seen in users of long wear contact lenses requires special communication with the microbiology laboratory	≤15 min at RT	Infection of the cornea requires urgent assessment and treatment by an ophthalmologist
Vitreous fluid	Vitreous fluid for bacterial cultures, fungal cultures	Suspicion of endophthalmitis with pain, loss of vision, increased secretions, and red eye	*S. aureus*, *S. epidermidis*, *P. aeruginosa*, viridans group streptococci, *H. influenzae*, *Bacillus* species, *Candida* species, fungi	Aspiration of vitreous fluid obtained at bedside or during surgical vitrectomy	Once and possibly repeated if clinically required	• Bacterial cultures • Fungal cultures	Positive results for a pathogen indicate a significant finding	Vitreal samples must be collected by an ophthalmologist and must be processed immediately in the microbiology laboratory	≤15 min at RT	Possible endophthalmitis requires urgent assessment and treatment by an ophthalmologist

Table 1-1: Specimen Selection, Collection, and Transport by Body Site *(continued)*

Gastrointestinal Samples										
General Category	Laboratory Test	Indications	Specific Microbes	Specimen	Frequency	Test Type	Interpretation	Advantages/ Disadvantages	Sample Transport	Key Points
Feces, rectal swab	• Microscopy • Stool culture • Toxin test	Diarrhea, food poisoning	• Bacterial pathogens: *Shigella* spp., *Salmonella* spp., *Vibrio cholerae*, *Escherichia coli*, *Campylobacter* spp. toxins of *Clostridium difficile*, *S. aureus*, *Bacillus cereus*, *Clostridium perfringens*, *Yersinia enterocolitica*, *Plesiomonas shigelloides* • Parasites: *Giardia intestinalis*, *Entamoeba histolytica*, *Dientamoeba fragilis*, *Cryptosporidium* spp. *Isospora belli*, *Sarcocystis hominis*, *Cyclospora cayetanensis*, *Encephalitozoon* spp. • Viruses: rotavirus, Norovirus	• 1 g of stool • At least 5 mL of diarrheal stool • If viruses are suspected, take 2–4 g of stool	Three consecutive specimens	• Culture, microscopy for ova and parasites, toxin test for *C. difficile* • Antigen detection by enzyme immunoassay (EIA) for *Giardia* and *Cryptosporidium* • PCR for norovirus and other viruses • PCR for *C. difficile* is now available and much more sensitive than EIA for toxins	• Fecal leukocyte examination recommended for differentiation between inflammatory and secretory diarrhea • Interpret carefully based on geographic location, season, and laboratory experience	Swabs not sensitive (recommended only for infants)	• Clean wide-mouthed container, unpreserved within 1 h, at RT • Holding medium within 24 h	• History of travel, specific food consumption • Fecal cultures are not performed for patients who stayed >3 days in hospital; test *C. difficile* in those patients
Gastric content	Gastric lavage	Tuberculosis in children	*Mycobacterium tuberculosis*	Introduce 50 mL chilled, sterile water through nasogastric tube	Once, in the morning	Acid-fast bacillus (AFB) smear, culture	Report all findings of culture and microscopy	This method is used when sputum is unavailable	Sterile container, ≤15 min, at RT	Method is used with children younger than 3 years

Table 1-1: Specimen Selection, Collection, and Transport by Body Site *(continued)*

Nervous System										
General Category	Laboratory Test	Indications	Specific Microbes	Specimen	Frequency	Test Type	Interpretation	Advantages/ Disadvantages	Sample Transport	Key Points
Cerebrospinal fluid (CSF)	• Microscopy • Culture	Meningitis and encephalitis	• *N. meningitidis, S. pneumoniae, S. agalactiae, L. monocytogenes,* Enterobacteria, *Leptospira* spp., *H. influenzae, S. aureus, M. tuberculosis* • Coxsackievirus, echovirus, poliovirus, HSV1 and HSV2, varicella zoster virus, flaviviruses, mumps virus, Bunyaviruses, Rubeola, lymphocytic choriomeningitis virus, adenoviruses • *Cryptococcus neoformans, Histoplasma capsulatum, Coccidioides immitis, Candida* spp., *Naegleria fowleri, Acanthamoeba* spp., *Angiostrongylus cantonensis*	Disinfect the skin with Povidine, iodine, or chlorhexidine gluconate and take 1–2 mL fluid into three tubes by lumbar puncture, or from ventricular shunt fluid	As clinically indicated	• Microscopy, culture, antigen detection, virus isolation • PCR for *N. meningitidis* and *S. pneumoniae* available in some labs and useful where culture fails • PCR for HSV and enteroviruses very sensitive	All findings from CSF are significant and should be reported immediately to clinician	Antigen tests are expensive and have low sensitivity	Sterile screw-capped tube, ≤15 min, at RT	• Obtain blood culture also • Collect sample before antimicrobial therapy • Patient age is important clue for possible agent

Table 1-1: Specimen Selection, Collection, and Transport by Body Site *(continued)*

Nervous System										
General Category	Laboratory Test	Indications	Specific Microbes	Specimen	Frequency	Test Type	Interpretation	Advantages/ Disadvantages	Sample Transport	Key Points
Cerebral tissue	Culture	Brain abscess	*Streptococcus* spp., *Peptostreptococcus* spp., *Porphyromonas* spp., *Bacteroides* spp., *Prevotella* spp., *Fusobacterium* spp., *Staphylococcus* spp., Enterobacteriaceae, *Burkholderia cepacia, S. pneumoniae, N. meningitidis, H. influenzae, Listeria monocytogenes, Haemophilus aphrophilus, Actinomyces* spp., *Nocardia* spp., Zygomycetes, *Mycobacterium* spp., *Naegleria* spp. (primary meningoencephalitis), *Acanthamoeba* spp., *Balamuthia mandrillaris* (granulomatous encephalitis)	• Brain biopsy specimen • Intraoperative specimen	As clinically indicated	• Culture, computed tomography • Specimen should be homogenized in sterile saline before plating	Brain abscess may rupture into subarachnoid space, producing severe meningitis	Swabs are not the optimum specimen to obtain purulent exudate	Transport under anaerobic conditions	Mainly occur as the result of direct extension from infections in surrounding areas

Urogenital Tract										
General Category	Laboratory Test	Indications	Specific Microbes	Specimen	Frequency	Test Type	Interpretation	Advantages/ Disadvantages	Sample Transport	Key Points
Urine	Urine culture	Urinary tract infections	*E. coli, Staphylococcus saprophyticus, Proteus* spp., *Klebsiella* spp., *Enterococcus* spp., *Pseudomonas* spp., *Candida* spp.	Urine (midstream, catheter, suprapubic)	One early morning specimen for symptomatic patients and two consecutive samples for asymptomatic patients	• Microscopy • Culture	Presence of single microbial isolate at >100,000 colony-forming unit (CFU)/mL is considered significant for all nosocomial infections (lower number applies to sexually active, symptomatic young women)	Do not culture indwelling Foley catheter tip or from indwelling catheter bags	Sterile container, ≤2 h, at RT	• Indicate whether or not the patient is symptomatic; pyuria is important consideration • Beware of asymptomatic bacteriuria in the elderly; in this case, pyuria also has very low specificity

Table 1-1: Specimen Selection, Collection, and Transport by Body Site *(continued)*

Urogenital Tract										
General Category	Laboratory Test	Indications	Specific Microbes	Specimen	Frequency	Test Type	Interpretation	Advantages/ Disadvantages	Sample Transport	Key Points
Genital, female	Culture	Chorioamnionitis, premature rupture of membranes >24 h	*Ureaplasma urealyticum*, *Mycoplasma hominis*, *Bacteroides* spp., *Gardnerella vaginalis*, *Streptococcus agalactiae*, *Peptostreptococcus* spp., *E. coli*, *Enterococcus* spp., *Fusobacterium* spp.	Amniotic fluid	Once	• Microscopy • Culture	Other analysis of amniotic fluid can reveal many aspects of the baby's genetic health	Swabbing of vaginal membranes is not acceptable	Anaerobic sterile tube, ≤2 h, at RT	Aspirate fluid via amniocentesis, or collect during Cesarean delivery
Genital, female	• Microscopy • Culture	Vaginitis, vulvovaginitis, vaginosis	• *Trichomonas vaginalis*, *Candida* spp., *Bacteroides* spp., *Prevotella bivia*, *Prevotella disiens*, *Prevotella* spp., *Actinomyces* spp., *Peptostreptococcus* spp. • *Gardnerella vaginalis*, *Mycoplasma hominis*	• Bartholin gland secretions • Vaginal discharge	As clinically indicated	• Microscopy • Culture	• High number of commensal flora makes vaginal specimens difficult to interpret • Bacterial vaginosis is diagnosed by microscopy	Pus from Bartholin gland can be collected with digital palpation; otherwise take by aspiration	Anaerobic transport system, ≤2 h, at RT	Do not process vaginal specimens for anaerobes because of the potential for contamination with commensal vaginal flora
Genital, female	Culture	Endometritis, cervicitis, pelvic inflammatory disease	*N. gonorrhoeae*, *C. trachomatis*, *S. agalactiae*, *Mycoplasma hominis*, HSV, *Bacteroides* spp.	• Endometrial tissue and secretions • Product of conception/ fetal tissue • Placenta • Membranes • Cervical secretions	As clinically indicated	• Swab • Culture	Gram stain can't be used effectively to detect *N. gonorrhoeae* in vaginal or cervical specimen	Likelihood for external contamination is high for cultures obtained through vagina	Anaerobic transport system, more than 1 mL, ≤2 h, at RT; cervical secretions in swab transport, ≤2 h, at RT	Visualize cervix with speculum and without lubricant; don't process lochia

Table 1-1: Specimen Selection, Collection, and Transport by Body Site *(continued)*

Urogenital Tract

General Category	Laboratory Test	Indications	Specific Microbes	Specimen	Frequency	Test Type	Interpretation	Advantages/ Disadvantages	Sample Transport	Key Points
Genital, male	• Gram stain • Cultures • Molecular probes	Urethritis, prostatitis, epididymitis	*N. gonorrhoeae, C. trachomatis, Ureaplasma urealyticum, E. coli*, other *Enterobacteriaceae, Pseudomonas* spp., *S. aureus, S. saprophyticus,* Enterococcus spp., *Trichomonas vaginalis*	• Insert a small swab 2–4 cm into urethral lumen, rotate 360 degrees, and leave it for 2 seconds • Prostate: cleanse meatus, massage prostate through rectum, collect fluid expressed from urethra on a sterile swab, or collect post prostate massage urine sample	As clinically indicated	• Urethral swabs • Immunologic tests • Culture	Positive stained smear diagnostic in a man with gonorrhea	Many specimens contaminated with normal skin or mucous membrane flora	Swab transport or sterile tube for more than 1 mL of specimen, ≤2 h, at RT	• The choice of swab is critical • Pathogens may be identified by quantitative culture of urine before and after massage

Hair, Nails, Skin

General Category	Laboratory Test	Indications	Specific Microbes	Specimen	Frequency	Test Type	Interpretation	Advantages/ Disadvantages	Sample Transport	Key Points
Hair, nails	• Microscopy • Culture	Dermatophytosis	*Trichophyton* spp., *Epidermophyton* spp., *Microsporum* spp., *Candida* spp., *Trichosporon* spp.	• Collect 10–12 hairs • Scrape infected nail area, or clip infected nail. • Collect hairs with intact shaft	As clinically indicated	• Hair • Scrapings	• Direct examination with potassium hydroxide, methylene blue, etc. • Report all findings from Saboro plate	Humidity in a closed system may cause the sample to be overgrown by bacteria	Clean container, ≤24 h, at RT	Culture for fungi may take several weeks
Skin	• Gram stain • Culture	Impetigo, erysipelas ecthyma, folliculitis, furunculus, and carbuncles; erythema migrans	*Streptococcus pyogenes* (Group A strep), *S. aureus, Borrelia burgdorferi, Trichophyton* spp., *Epidermophyton* spp., *Microsporum* spp., *Candida* spp., *Malassezia* spp., *Sporothrix schenckii*	Skin sample	• Once • Repeat as needed	Swabs, biopsy, or aspirate aseptically collected	Presence of leukocytes represents appropriate specimen	High likelihood of contamination	Clean container, ≤2 h, at RT	The skin surface should be disinfected with 70% alcohol

Table 1-1: Specimen Selection, Collection, and Transport by Body Site *(continued)*

Hair, Nails, Skin

General Category	Laboratory Test	Indications	Specific Microbes	Specimen	Frequency	Test Type	Interpretation	Advantages/ Disadvantages	Sample Transport	Key Points
Skin, wounds	• Microscopy • Culture	Acute wound infections, chronic wound infections, cellulitis, necrotizing fasciitis, Fournier's gangrene	Aerobic and facultative microorganism: Coagulase-negative staphylococci, *S. aureus*, beta-hemolytic streptococci, *Enterococcus* spp., *Streptococcus viridans* group, *Corynebacterium* spp., *Bacillus cereus*, *E. coli*, *Serratia* spp., *Klebsiella* spp., *Enterobacter* spp., Citrobacter spp., *Morganella morganii*, *Providencia stuartii*, *Proteus* spp., *Pseudomonas aeruginosa*, *Acinetobacter baumannii*, *S. maltophilia*, Anaerobic bacteria: *Peptostreptococcus* spp., *Clostridium* spp., *Bacteroides fragilis* group, *Prevotella* spp., etc.	• Cutaneous abscesses, postsurgical wounds, bites, decubitus ulcer, skin abscess, burns, soft tissues • Representative specimen is taken from advancing margin of the lesion • Take abscess specimen by aspiration	• Once • Repeat as needed	• Aspirate • Swab	Gram stain should assess the quality of sample	• Tissue or aspirate is always superior to swab specimen • If swab must be used, collect two swabs	Swab transport system or anaerobic transport system, ≤2 h, at RT	Attention to skin decontamination is critical

References

Allen S, Procop G, Schreckenberger P. Guidelines for the collection, transport, processing, analysis, and reporting of cultures from specific specimen sources. In: Winn WC, Koneman EE, eds. *Koneman's Color Atlas and Textbook of Diagnostic Microbiology*, 6th ed. Philadelphia: Lippincott Williams & Wilkins, 2006:68-105.

Diekema DJ, Pfaller MA. Infection control epidemiology and clinical microbiology. In: Murray PR, ed. *Manual of Clinical Microbiology*, 9th ed. Washington, DC: ASM, 2007:118-129.

Jarvis WR, Brachman PS, Bennett JV. The role of the laboratory in control of healthcare-associated infections. In: *Bennett & Brachman's Hospital Infections*, 5th ed. Philadelphia: Lippincott Williams & Wilkins, 2007:121-150.

Kalenić S, Budimir A. The role of microbiology laboratory in healthcare-associated infection prevention. *Int J Infect Control* 2009;5(2).

Miller M, Krisher K, Holms H. General principles of specimen collection and handling. In: Murray PR, ed. *Manual of Clinical Microbiology*, 9th ed. Washington, DC: ASM, 2007:43-55.

Murray PR, Witebsky FG. The clinician and the microbiology laboratory. In: Mandell GL, ed. *Mandell, Douglas, and Bennett's Principles and Practice of Infectious Diseases*, 7th ed. Philadelphia: Churchill Livingstone, 2010:233-266.

Peterson LR, Hamilton JD, Baron EJ, et al. Role of clinical microbiology laboratory in the management and control of infectious diseases and the delivery of health care. *Clin Infect Dis* 2001;32:605-611.

Poutanen SM, Tompkins LS. Molecular methods in nosocomial epidemiology. In: Wenzel RP, ed. *Prevention and Control of Nosocomial Infections*, 4th ed. Philadelphia: Lippincott, Williams & Wilkins, 2003:481-499.

Roberts L. Specimen collection and processing. In: Mahon C, Lehman DC, Manuselis G, eds. *Textbook of Diagnostic Microbiology*, 4th ed. St. Louis: Saunders, 2011:111-126.

Stratton IV CW, Greene JN. Role of the microbiology laboratory in hospital epidemiology and infection control. In: Mayhall CG, ed. *Hospital Epidemiology and Infection Control*, 3rd ed. Philadelphia: Lippincott Williams & Wilkins, 2004:1809-1825.

Van Eldere J. Changing needs, opportunities, and constraints for the 21st century microbiology laboratory. *Clin Microbiol Infect* 2005;11(Suppl 1): 15-18.

Chapter 2

Cultures and Gram stains

Kathy Aureden, MS, MT(ASCP)SI, CIC

Additional Contributors:
Sallie Jo Rivera, RN, MSN, CIC
Susan Wagoner, BS, MT(ASCP)SM

Clinical and surveillance specimens are submitted to the clinical laboratory for quick and accurate detection of significant microbes that may be involved in an infectious disease process. Laboratory specialties for detection of clinically important and disease-causing microbes (pathogens) include microbiology, virology, parasitology, mycology (fungi), mycobacteriology, surgical pathology, and molecular diagnostics.

This chapter reviews laboratory tests utilizing microscopy (routine and special staining procedures) and microbiological cultures (see Table 2-2). It is very important to select the appropriate specimen to be submitted, ensure appropriate timing of collection, and utilize the correct method of collection to maximize recovery of potential pathogen(s) for diagnosis of an infectious process. Please refer to Chapter 1, Specimen Collection and Transport, for more information regarding these factors.

No single laboratory test is available that permits isolation of all possible pathogens. Clinical information, such as tentative diagnosis and suspected type of infection, aids in the selection of the proper media and incubation conditions for the isolation of the suspected pathogens. The specimen type will determine other culture requirements for the suspected pathogen(s) as outlined in the facility's laboratory protocol. For example, a stool sent for bacterial culture is appropriate when bacterial gastroenteritis (e.g., shigellosis, *Campylobacter* infection, typhoid fever) is suspected. A stool specimen order for ova and parasites is submitted for the detection of amebiasis, giardiasis, or intestinal parasitic "worms." An order for norovirus polymerase chain reaction (PCR) is indicated when the presence of this specific virus in a stool specimen is clinically relevant.

Important considerations regarding specimens and types of cultures
- Specimens for bacterial and fungal culture must be collected prior to initiation of antimicrobial therapy. This will ensure that organisms present in the specimen are viable for growth in culture.
- A culture result can only accurately depict the infectious process if the specimen is adequate. Laboratory collection manuals provide specific specimen collection directions to ensure an optimal specimen.
- A sufficient quantity of specimen must be submitted to ensure that all of the requested tests can be performed.
- The process of "splitting" a specimen for multiple tests must be done in a way that does not contaminate or compromise the specimen prior to setting up cultures.

Surveillance cultures require specimens from patient sites, and occasionally from environmental sites, that are known to be implicated as an ongoing source of the organism in question, as may be the case for methicillin-resistant *Staphylococcus aureus* (MRSA), vancomycin-resistant enterococci (VRE), *Acinetobacter*, and other organisms. When doing surveillance cultures of patients, knowledge of the usual sites of colonization or infection will determine specimen type. Environmental surveillance cultures require knowledge about preferred sites in which the organism persists. Surveillance cultures may be considered necessary based on an outbreak analysis or may be indicated by the facility's ongoing infection prevention risk assessment. In either case, the infection preventionist must define a surveillance plan and a standardized process consistent with evidence-based, expert guidance from the Centers for Disease Control and Prevention (CDC) and other recognized professional organizations when implementing a surveillance culture intervention or program. The reader is referred to the Healthcare Infection Control Practices Advisory Committee's 2006 *Management of Multidrug-resistant Organisms in Healthcare Settings* guideline for evidence-based guidance on this topic.

Microscopy Defined and Described

Microscopy is the science of observing images of objects (e.g., cells, microbes) that cannot be seen by the unaided eye. The most common type of microscopy performed in the microbiology lab is bright-field microscopy, in which visible light is used to illuminate a magnified image of an object. In order for the object to be best observed, as well as provide information about the structural and physiologic makeup of the cell, chemicals with well-known characteristics in staining (coloring) cells are used.

The most widely used stain in the microbiology laboratory is the Gram stain, which is used to make visible and, in certain well-defined ways, to differentiate kinds of bacteria and cells (e.g., white blood cells). The Gram stain includes four chemicals, each providing a crucial step in the process that distinguishes a Gram-positive (purple staining) cell from a Gram-negative (pink/red staining) cell (see Figure 2-1). A Gram stain of a specimen, when appropriate, can provide immediate information about an infectious process. Organisms isolated from culture are Gram stained to determine which additional tests must be done to quickly and accurately identify the organism and provide a culture result.

Figure 2-1: Gram stain

1. Add crystal violet dye to thin smear of specimen or bacterial cell mixture dried onto a microscope slide to stain cells purple.
2. Add Gram's iodine solution (mordant) to form a large complex between the crystal violet and iodine.
3. Add decolorizer (ethyl alcohol/acetone)—the crystal violet iodine complex is trapped in a Gram-positive cell but can escape from a Gram-negative cell (related to makeup of the cell outer membrane).
4. Add counterstain (safranin), which stains a decolorized Gram-negative cell red but does not affect the purple color of the Gram-positive cells that were not decolonized in previous step.

Note: Gram stain results always give the staining characteristic plus the morphologic shape of the microbe.
  Gram-negative bacillus (bacilli = plural), AKA Gram-negative rod, refers to pink, cylindrically-shaped microbes.
  Gram-positive bacillus (bacilli = plural), AKA Gram-positive rod, refers to purple, cylindrically-shaped microbes.
  Gram-negative coccus (cocci = plural) refers to pink, spherically-shaped microbes.
  Gram-positive coccus (cocci = plural) refers to purple, spherically-shaped microbes.

Other stains and microscopy techniques are used by laboratory professionals to characterize specific organisms or tissues that may contain pathogens, including wet preps, direct and indirect immunofluorescence, dark field microscopy, acid fast stains, and electron microscopy. Table 2-1 provides an overview of Gram stain terminology and results.

Microbial Cultures Defined and Described

A microbiologic culture is a laboratory technique used to grow (cultivate) bacteria and yeast. A culture of a clinical specimen can yield polymicrobial growth (more than one type of bacteria cultivated in culture), pure culture (single bacterial strain cultivated in culture), or no growth (no bacteria recovered from clinical specimen).

Identification of the bacteria or yeast grown in culture results in a genus and species designation written in italics (e.g., *S. aureus*—genus first, species second). On occasion, and if sufficiently significant for identification purposes, microbes are identified by genus only (e.g., *Staphylococcus* sp., where sp. stands for species, plural spp.) signifying that the isolate is a member of the group referred to as staphylococci; or genus plus a laboratory distinguishing characteristic (e.g., coagulase negative *Staphylococcus*).

When clinically significant, the growth on cultures may be quantified or semiquantified. An example of a quantified culture result is typical in urine cultures (e.g., 50,000 colony-forming units [CFU] *Escherichia coli*). An example of a semiquantitative result is typical in throat culture (e.g., heavy growth Group A *Streptococcus pyogenes*). Some cultures do not require a quantitative result (e.g., blood culture positive for *Streptococcus pneumoniae*).

Microbiology Techniques

Laboratory professionals perform many tests to identify the microbes isolated in cultures and to determine the antimicrobial susceptibilities for clinically significant microbes. It is outside the scope of this chapter to review these techniques in depth, so a brief synopsis of bacterial culture techniques and aids are provided here.

Growth media, broth (liquid), or agar (solid or semisolid) that provide nutrients microbes required for growth

- Basic media: nonselective, most organisms will grow (e.g., blood agar, BHI broth, chocolate agar), colony morphology is part of the identifying workup for bacteria grown on solid media (agar)
- Selective media: incorporates antibiotics or inhibitory chemicals to inhibit growth of unwanted type of bacteria and/or preferentially encourage growth of significant bacteria
- Different media: incorporates dyes or chemicals (usually carbohydrates) that provide preliminary organism identification
- Indicator (e.g., chromagenic) media: incorporates indicator(s) that permits identification of certain significant bacteria based on uptake of a dye or development of a color

Optimal incubation parameters are provided as required by different bacteria

- Temperature requirements
- Nutrient requirements
- Incubation atmosphere (O_2, CO_2, etc.) requirements
- Time required for sufficient growth and further testing; 24 to 48 hours for indigenous flora and many microbial pathogens, 4 to 6 weeks for *Mycobacterium tuberculosis*, etc.
- Additional time required for susceptibility testing of isolates recovered from culture (24 to 48 hours)

Differential Testing

- Tests of biochemical responses and carbohydrate fermentation for organism identification
- Tests for microbe specific enzymes, and toxins (e.g., coagulase test, catalase test)
- Motility tests
- Germ tube test (yeast)
- Direct fluorescent antibody tests for specific bacteria
- Latex agglutination (e.g., determining streptococci groups; group A = *Streptococcus pyogenes*, group B = *Streptococcus agalactiae*, etc.)

Special Methods

Molecular testing methodologies have greatly enhanced the speed, specificity, and sensitivity of tests for clinically significant microbes. Examples of molecular testing methods are PCR, pulse field gel electrophoresis, Western blot assay, enzyme linked immunoassays, and molecular genotypic assays.

Final Note

Infection preventionists and clinical providers rely greatly on the microbiology laboratory for information crucial to infection prevention interventions and for clinical decision making. The work of the microbiology laboratory is instrumental in surveillance programs for detecting emerging significant and multidrug resistant pathogens, public health or facility outbreaks, and potential bioterrorism events. A strong, ongoing partnership between microbiology laboratory professionals and infection preventionists should remain a top priority in all infection prevention programs to ensure maximum patient safety and positive patient outcomes.

Table 2-1: Gram Stain Terminology and Results

Stain Type and Prep Time	Organism Morphology and Staining Characteristics	Specific Microbe Examples (not all-inclusive)	Key Points and Clarifications
Bright Field Microscopy			
Gram stain: 3 minutes	Gram-positive cocci "in chains"	Group A, B, C, G *Streptococcus* spp., *Enterococcus*, *Peptostreptococcus*, etc.	• Coccus (plural, cocci) is spherical shape • Clusters of cocci of staphylococci can be referred to as "grape-like" (note: staphyle from Greek for "cluster of grapes")
	Gram-positive cocci "in pairs" (diplococci)	*Streptococcus pneumoniae*, *Enterococcus* (pairs, or chains), *Micrococcus* (tetrad)	"Bacillus" is from Latin baculum meaning rod (e.g., Gram-negative bacillus AKA Gram-negative rod)
	Gram-positive cocci "in clusters"	*Staphylococcus* spp. (MRSA, MSSA, *S. epidermidis*, other staphylococci), diphtheroids (*Corynebacteria* spp.)	• Gram-positive = purple • Gram-negative = pink
	Gram-positive rods with or without endospores	*Clostridium* spp., *Bacillus* spp., *Listeria*, pleomorphic, coryneform bacteria (e.g., diphtheroids)	Gram variable organisms may appear as variably purple or partly pink (not uniformly stained)
	Gram variable rods	*Bacillus* spp., *Lactobacillus* spp.	Gram-positive rods with internal spores (endospores) do not stain where the spore is located within the organism
	Gram-negative cocci	*Neisseria* (pairs "diplococci"), *Kingella*	Coccobacillary means rounded rod shaped (e.g., *Acinetobacter* has coccobacillus shape)
	Gram-negative rods	Enterobacteriaceae (*E. coli*, *Enterobacter*, *Klebsiella*, etc.), environmental Gram-negative rods (*Pseudomonas*, *Acinetobacter*, etc.), anaerobic Gram-negative rods (*Bacteroides*, *Fusobacteria*, *Prevotella*), others	• Diplo = one pair • Tetrad = two pairs in a square • Pleomorphic means nonuniform shape • Bipolar "safety pin" stain (consider *Yersinia* or *Burkholderia*)
	Spirochetes	*Treponema*, *Borrelia*, *Leptospira*	• Gram stain is not usually effective for detection of spirochetes • May be detected by darkfield or fluorescent microscopy
	Yeast and fungi	*Candida* spp., *Cryptococcus*, *Aspergillus*, *Blastomyces*, *Coccidioides*	• Special stains may be used (Gram stain not always effective) • Larger than bacteria, budding yeast and/or branching hyphae may be described
Acid fast stain: ≤ 2 hours	Detects "acid fast" and "partially acid fast" bacteria	Mycobacteria, *Nocardia*, *Cryptosporidium*	• Used for organisms that cannot be stained using Gram stain • Longer staining process • Methods: Ziehl-Neelsen, Kinyoun techniques
Wet mount: 1 minute	No stain used, check for fungi or parasites; check for motile organisms	*Trichomonas*, fungal hyphae, or yeast	Useful in vaginal specimens to detect trichomas, clue cells typical of *Gardnerella vaginalis* (vaginal epithelial cells with many adherent bacteria)
Potassium hydroxide (KOH) prep: 5–10 minutes	Direct exam for fungi	*Trichophyton*, *Microsporum* (ringworm, tinea, etc.)	Useful in skin and nail scrapings, body fluids
Wright-Giemsa stain: 10–60 minutes	Detect parasites in blood smear	*Plasmodium* spp. (malaria), *Babesia*, *Leishmania*, *Trypanosoma*, some fungi in tissue specimen	Malarial forms detected on this stain may be diagnostic (may be able to determine species type)
Periodic acid-Schiff (PAS): 60 minutes	Fungal yeast and hyphal forms in tissue specimen	Most fungi are stained by this method	

Table 2-1: Gram Stain Terminology and Results *(continued)*

Stain Type and Prep Time	Organism Morphology and Staining Characteristics	Specific Microbe Examples (not all-inclusive)	Key Points and Clarifications
India ink	Encapsulated yeast	*Cryptococcus* spp.	• "Halo effect" around organism • Useful test on spinal fluid, other body fluids
Trichrome	Parasites in stool	*Giardia, Entamoeba, Endolimax*	• Detects protozoan cysts, eggs, trophozoites
Microscopy–Other			
Darkfield microscopy	Motile forms of bacteria and other cells	Spirochetes, sperm, protozoa	• Special microscope lens and filter system • Bright organisms seen against a black background
Fluorescent microscopy	Fluorescent dye linked to antibody specific to organism of interest	Direct antibody tests and indirect antibody tests (technique specific) to detect antigen of organism, cell, etc.	• Special microscope lens and filter system • Fluorescing organisms seen against a black background • Color is specific to fluorescent dye used (often fluorescent green or red)

Table 2-2: Overview of Cultures and Gram Stains

General Category	Laboratory Test	Indications	Specific Microbes	Specimen	Frequency	Test Type	Interpretation	Advantages/ Disadvantages	Key Points
Microbiology: Culture and sensitivity for clinical management of patient condition	Blood culture	Clinical sepsis, fever of unknown origin, pneumonia, suspected catheter-related bloodstream infection, subacute or acute bacterial endocarditis, urosepsis, neonatal sepsis	Aerobic and anaerobic Gram-positive cocci (e.g., *Streptococcus*, *Staphylococcus*), Gram-positive rods (*Bacillus*), Gram-negative rods (e.g., *Escherichia coli*, *Pseudomonas*), Gram-negative cocci (e.g., *Neisseria*), mycobacteria, yeast, other fungi, others	• Blood obtained via aseptic venipuncture • Requires immediate dispensing into bottle containing liquid media provided by laboratory • Collection volume critical • One set = two bottles (aerobe and anaerobe) obtained multiple different times to assess possibility of contaminant and to help assess line infections	For central line-associated bloodstream infections, surveillance criteria require two sets drawn within 2 days of each other when the organism is common skin flora	• Routine culture and sensitivity • Automated blood culture system • Gram stain of positive bottles • Polymerase chain reaction (PCR) testing • Note that positive bottles are flagged by instrument, Gram stain then done and blood from bottle is cultured on agar media	• Pathogen from one or more bottles indicates infection related to device or procedure (e.g., sepsis, bacteremia, or candidemia) • Other infection (pneumonia, urinary tract infection [UTI], etc.)	• Important clinical significance when pathogen is recovered • Contamination with skin flora during collection can lead to "false positive" • Identification and antibiotic susceptibility typically resulted within 3–5 days	• Gram stain results aid in early indication of possible pathogens • Aerobes and anaerobes can be isolated; organism identification and antibiotic susceptibility pattern in final result • Specimen collection technique critical to prevent contamination of specimen—cleanse skin site using chlorhexidine gluconate (CHG) and disinfect top of collection bottle with an antiseptic product before collecting specimen
	Cerebral spinal fluid (CSF) culture	Meningitis, encephalitis, post-procedures accessing epidural space or spinal canal, neonatal sepsis	*Streptococcus pneumoniae*, *Neisseria meningitidis*, *Haemophilus influenzae*, Group B *Streptococcus*, especially in neonates, *S. aureus*, *Cryptococcus* fungi, mycobacteria, viral pathogens such as West Nile virus (WNV), Eastern equine encephalitis virus (EEE), varicella, herpes, prions	• CSF • Note that if prion disease is a consideration, special handling of used equipment and follow-up of unanticipated exposures is necessary	Acute illness onset; chronic condition (e.g., prion disease or multiple sclerosis)	• Bacterial culture and Gram stain • Viral culture • Cryptococcals antigen • Fungal culture • PCR test for specific pathogens	Gram stain may reveal Gram-positive diplococcus (*S. pneumoniae*), Gram-negative diplococcus (*Neisseria meningitidis*), small Gram-negative rods (*Haemophilus*), Gram-positive cocci in chains (*Streptococcus*) or clusters (*Staphylococcus*), Gram-positive rods (*Listeria*), yeast (*Candida* or *Cryptococcus*)		• Test CSF for cell count, glucose, protein, and lactic acid (see below) • Tests for prion disease require special attention and may not be readily available • Special tests are required if differential diagnosis and include multiple sclerosis (e.g., CSF oligoclonal bands and myelin basic protein)

Table 2-2: Overview of Cultures and Gram Stains (*continued*)

General Category	Laboratory Test	Indications	Specific Microbes	Specimen	Frequency	Test Type	Interpretation	Advantages/ Disadvantages	Key Points
Microbiology: Culture and sensitivity for clinical management of patient condition (*continued*)	CSF cell count and chemistry; additional laboratory tests	Meningitis, encephalitis, post-procedures accessing epidural space or spinal canal, neonatal sepsis	*Streptococcus pneumoniae, Neisseria meningitidis, Haemophilus influenzae*, Group B *Streptococcus*, especially in neonates, *S. aureus, Cryptococcus* fungi, mycobacteria, viral pathogens such as West Nile virus (WNV), Eastern equine encephalitis virus (EEE), varicella, herpes, prions	• CSF • Note that if prion disease is a consideration, special handling of used equipment and follow-up of unanticipated exposures is necessary	Acute illness onset; chronic condition (e.g., prion disease or multiple sclerosis)	• Hematology • Chemistry	• Gram stain: presence of >5 white blood cells (WBCs) in non-bloody specimen • Predominant neutrophils (segs) common in bacterial disease • Predominant lymphocytes common in viral disease • Eosinophils ($>10/mm^3$) in parasitic meningitis (e.g., *Angiostrongylus*) and fungal meningitis (e.g., *Coccidioides*)		• In addition to CSF culture: presence of WBCs (neutrophils or lymphocytes), increase in protein and decrease in glucose may be associated with bacterial meningitis • Neutrophils (segs) and normal glucose may be associated with early viral (enterovirus, WNV, EEE, St. Louis encephalitis) • Lymphocytes and normal glucose may be associated with viral • Lymphocytes present with low glucose may be associated with tuberculosis (TB), fungal, tumor
	Body fluid culture	Fluid aspirated from joint or organ space	Aerobic and anaerobic bacteria, fungi, mycobacteria, and other acid-fast bacilli (AFB)	• Knee, hip, or other joint fluid • Pleural fluid • Pericardial fluid • Peritoneal (ascites)	Acute illness onset; chronic condition complication	• Aerobic and anaerobic culture • Fungal culture • AFB culture	Gram stain positive for WBCs, bacteria, yeast can be significant for infection; WBCs may only indicate noninfectious inflammation	• Quick aid to treatment if Gram stain is positive for bacteria • If bacterial, identification and antibiotic susceptibility typically resulted within 3–5 days	If organisms that cannot be cultured are suspected, order organism-specific tests; additional laboratory tests include body fluid protein, glucose, other stains

Table 2-2: Overview of Cultures and Gram Stains (*continued*)

General Category	Laboratory Test	Indications	Specific Microbes	Specimen	Frequency	Test Type	Interpretation	Advantages/ Disadvantages	Key Points
Microbiology: Culture and sensitivity for clinical management of patient condition (*continued*)	Lower respiratory culture	Lower respiratory infection (LRI) tracheobronchitis, pneumonia, empyema, opportunistic infections of the lower respiratory tract in immunosuppressed patients	Aerobic and anaerobic bacteria including *Streptococcus pneumoniae, Klebsiella pneumoniae, Staphylococcus aureus, Mycobacterium tuberculosis* and other AFB, *Nocardia* and *Actinomyces, Histoplasma, Blastomyces, Coccidioides, Mycoplasma,* viral pathogens, *Pneumocystis,* others	• Sputum • Induced sputum • Bronchoscopy (lavage, brush biopsy, etc.)	Acute illness (bacterial, viral); chronic illness (some fungal, opportunistic, mycobacterial, and parasitic etiologies)	• Gram stain • Routine culture • Susceptibility • Blood culture • Fungal culture • AFB/mycobacterial stain and culture • Viral culture • PCR testing for specific pathogen	• Gram stain of sterile site specimen can be significant • On Gram stain of sputum, if 25 epithelial cells/HPF, specimen is inadequate for diagnostic purposes • Bacteria in blood culture can be accurate indicator of microbial etiology of infection • Pathogens isolated from adequate lower respiratory infections are significant • Environmental organisms isolated from specimens in patients on ventilator may be clinically significant	• Organism cultured from blood can be significant in pneumonia • Bronchoscopy specimen is preferred over sputum as upper respiratory normal flora in culture can confound assessment of clinical picture • Some lower respiratory pathogens have very specific culture requirements often only available at reference labs • Some pathogens (e.g., mycobacteria, *Nocardia,* and *Actinomyces,* fungal pathogens) require weeks and sometimes months to cultivate and identify	• If organisms that cannot be cultured are suspected, order organism-specific tests • Additional stains may be appropriate (e.g., AFB, PAS, others) • Bacteria aspirated from throat (normal flora) may cause pneumonia or LRI but may also be contaminants from nonsterile specimen collection via upper respiratory tract
	Upper respiratory culture	Throat infection, nasal colonization, or abscess	Group A *Streptococcus* (*Streptococcus pyogenes*), *Staphylococcus aureus,* influenza, *Candida, Haemophilus influenzae* (children), *Neisseria meningitidis* carriers, others	• Throat swab • Anterior nares swab • Nasopharyngeal aspirate	Acute upper respiratory illness, sinusitis, infection prevention surveillance	Culture or rapid point of care (POC) test for Group A strep and influenza	• Known respiratory pathogens identified in culture or by POC test is clinically significant • "Normal throat flora" is resulted as such in culture • Gram stain is generally not helpful due to presence of normal flora	• Specimen easy to obtain • POC test results available quickly • POC test (waived test) often done in satellite labs or doctor's offices	• POC tests for Group A strep and influenza are often less sensitive • Negative result may be followed up by culture or other confirmatory test

Table 2-2: Overview of Cultures and Gram Stains (continued)

General Category	Laboratory Test	Indications	Specific Microbes	Specimen	Frequency	Test Type	Interpretation	Advantages/ Disadvantages	Key Points
Microbiology: Culture and sensitivity for clinical management of patient condition *(continued)*	Other tests for upper respiratory infection	Whooping cough, sore throat, parotitis, coughing, illness	*Bordetella pertussis*, mumps, respiratory syncytial virus (RSV), influenza, other bacterial and viral agents	Nasopharyngeal collection (swab or aspirate)	Acute illness	• POC test • PCR • Direct fluorescent antibody (DFA) • Viral culture	Negative POC test result may be followed up by confirmatory test	• Nasopharyngeal collection more invasive • Special transport media based on microbe suspected may be required	Specimen collection technique critical to recovery of organisms—ensure nasopharyngeal technique used (See Chapter 8 for antibody tests)
	Urinary tract culture	UTI including bladder or kidney infection; kidney stones in urinary tract are sometimes associated with bacteriuria (bacteria in urine) with or without symptoms of infection	*E. coli*, *Enterobacter*, *Klebsiella*, *Morganella*, *Citrobacter*, *Proteus*, *Pseudomonas*, *Serratia*, *Enterococcus* spp., *Staphylococcus* spp., *Candida* spp., others	Specimen obtained by "clean catch" or aseptic collection of urinary catheter	Acute illness, urologic condition	Quantitative culture and susceptibility	• Symptomatic UTI colony count >100,000 CFU/mL with no more than 2 species is clinically significant • Or 1000 – 100,000 CFU with pyuria per NHSN criteria • Urinalysis frequently of additional help (See Chapter 9)	Clinical assessment differentiates symptomatic UTI from asymptomatic bacteriuria	• Specimen collection technique and prompt delivery to microbiology to ensure specimen integrity • Do not routinely order culture in patients with urinary catheter unless UTI is suspected by clinician • DO NOT culture urinary catheter tips
	Wounds and abscess culture	Skin and soft tissue infections, cellulitis, necrotizing fasciitis	*Staphylococci*, *Streptococcus* spp., Gram-negative bacteria, yeast, and fungi	• Aseptically obtained abscess aspiration or tissue • Swab of advancing margin of base of wound after cleansing outer portion of wound	Acute infection	• Culture and Gram stain • Other culture types per clinical request	Presence of organisms correlated with symptoms and clinical status	Gram stain of specimen aseptically obtained from wound bed can direct empiric treatment before culture results	• Specimen collection technique important for actual organism recovery • Skin flora contamination possible
	Surgical site infection (SSI) cultures	SSI symptoms associated with skin incision, deep tissue, or organ space surgical site	Surgical site pathogens may include normal skin, respiratory or intestinal flora, environmental microbes, fungus, mycobacteria, *Nocardia*, *Actinomyces*, anaerobic microbes, others	• Aseptically obtained abscess aspiration or tissue • Swab of advancing margin of base of wound after cleansing outer portion of wound • Computed tomography (CT)-guided specimen collection, surgical debridement specimen	Acute illness or acute symptoms	Routine culture and Gram stain	Presence of organisms is correlated with symptoms and clinical status	Gram stain of specimen aseptically obtained from surgical site can direct empiric treatment before culture results	See CDC and NHSN surveillance criteria for additional information regarding SSI criteria and designations

Table 2-2: Overview of Cultures and Gram Stains *(continued)*

General Category	Laboratory Test	Indications	Specific Microbes	Specimen	Frequency	Test Type	Interpretation	Advantages/ Disadvantages	Key Points
Microbiology: Culture and sensitivity for clinical management of patient condition *(continued)*	Gastrointestinal (GI) tract infections	GI symptoms per infectious etiology	*Salmonella, Shigella, Campylobacter, Giardia, Vibrio, Yersinia, Clostridium difficile* or its toxins, norovirus, rotavirus, *Entamoeba, Giardia, Cryptosporidium*, ova from parasitic "worms," tapeworm (whole or segments), nematodes, trematodes (flatworms), yeast, alterations in normal flora, others	• Stool, colonic washings • Occasionally emesis specimen, blood, or urine	Acute illness, when diarrheal specimen can be obtained	• Routine culture • Ova and parasite test • PCR tests • Gross exam for intestinal worms (including worm segments)	Presence of pathogens, ova and/or parasites, toxins correlated with GI symptoms	• Ova and parasite test • PCR and toxin tests may be available same day • Culture results often available within 48 hours	• Diarrheal stool specimen indicates active condition and is required when testing for *C. difficile* toxin • Urine and blood may also be positive for *Salmonella* or *Shigella* • Copious stool flora requires selective and enhanced media for isolation of pathogens
	Genital infections	Symptoms of genital infection	*Candida* spp. ("yeast"), *Gardnerella vaginalis* (bacterial vaginosis), *Trichomonas*			• Culture • PCR • Gram stain • Wet mount	• Motile flagellar protozoan, size of a **WBC** = *Trichomonas* • Budding cells smaller than an **RBC** = yeast +/- pseudohyphae • Clue cells = epithelial cells with adherent bacteria		• *Candida* can be detected in culture or wet prep • *Trichomonas* is detected in wet prep • *Gardnerella vaginalis* can be detected in wet prep or Gram stain (clue cells)
		Sexually transmitted disease testing per clinical assessment	*Neisseria gonorrhoeae, Trichomonas, Chlamydia trachomatis*				Gram-negative diplococci suggests *N. gonorrhoeae*		PCR test is used for *Chlamydia trachomatis* (Gram-negative intracellular parasite and not readily grown in culture) PCR or culture can detect *N. gonorrhoeae*
			Treponema pallidum (syphilis)						Motile spirochete that may be detected in a specimen using darkfield microscopy; however, is generally tested for by serologies (immune response) including RPR (nonspecific) and FTA, TPA, etc. (specific)

Table 2-2: Overview of Cultures and Gram Stains (*continued*)

General Category	Laboratory Test	Indications	Specific Microbes	Specimen	Frequency	Test Type	Interpretation	Advantages/ Disadvantages	Key Points
Microbiology: Culture and sensitivity for clinical management of patient condition (*continued*)	Maternal surveillance cultures for clinical management	Pregnancy, maternal issues	Group B *Streptococcus* (GBS)	For GBS, lower vaginal and/or rectal swab	Obtain 1 specimen at 35–37 weeks	Culture or PCR	Presence of GBS—clinicians follow CDC guidelines	• Timing during pregnancy is important • Labor occurring prior to screening tests results in alternate clinical options per CDC guidelines	• PCR is faster than culture when test is ordered STAT in a laboring woman with no prior testing • GBS in urine can be a marker for vaginal GBS colonization
			Hepatitis B and HIV	Blood test					Serologic test for immune status and/or active infection
Microbiology: Culture for infection prevention and control purposes	MRSA surveillance cultures; other surveillance cultures per infection prevention (IP) policies or during outbreak situations	Annual, ongoing surveillance per infection prevention risk assessment, other surveillance cultures per IP policies	MRSA, VISA/VRSA (vancomycin-intermediate or resistant *S.aureus*); other organisms per IP risk assessment, may include multidrug-resistant *Acinetobacter, Pseudomonas, Stenotrophomonas,* VRE, ESBL Gram-negative rods, carbapenemase-resistant Gram-negative rods (including KPC, CBE, NDM-1), drug resistant *Streptococcus pneumoniae, Neisseria gonorrhoeae,* other emerging pathogens	MRSA surveillance via nasal swab at minimum, other sites as appropriate for organism of interest	Surveillance for colonization; per IP policy	• Routine culture • Chromogenic agar • PCR	Colonization assumed if organism is detected	Surveillance cultures ordered for IP purposes (e.g., transmission based precautions, patient risk groups, outbreaks, etc.)	• Surveillance cultures not routinely done for clinical management of patient unless medically indicated • Surveillance cultures are used for patient placement purposes and for decisions on discontinuing precautions • Note: surveillance cultures for staff colonization not routinely indicated unless staff are implicated in cluster/outbreak

Table 2-2: Overview of Cultures and Gram Stains *(continued)*

General Category	Laboratory Test	Indications	Specific Microbes	Specimen	Frequency	Test Type	Interpretation	Advantages/ Disadvantages	Key Points
Microbiology: Culture for infection prevention and control purposes *(continued)*	Other surveillance situations	Outbreak or increased incidence in population, unit, or facility; surveillance as indicated per IP risk assessment	Emerging pathogens, significant pathogen cluster, outbreak investigation, possible bioterrorism event	Specimen determined by normal colonization site of organism of interest and presence of patient tubes or lines	Per IP policy for surveillance cultures	• Routine culture • Chromogenic or other specialty agars • PCR • Sensitivity if indicated for microbe identification • Genotypic testing if indicated in outbreak investigation	Presence of organism indicates colonization unless symptoms of upper respiratory infection are present and/or infection is suspected	• Surveillance cultures ordered for infection prevention purposes per infection prevention risk assessment • Cultures not done for medical management of patient	• Outbreak surveillance cultures aids in characterization and control of outbreak • Annual infection prevention risk assessment determines routine surveillance culture criteria • Bioterrorism events—special considerations and laboratory requirements, obtain guidance from public health department and CDC

References

Centers for Disease Control and Prevention. *Catheter-associated urinary tract infection (CAUTI) event.* Centers for Disease Control and Prevention. 2009. Available at: http://www.cdc.gov/nhsn/pdfs/pscManual/7pscCAUTIcurrent.pdf. Accessed December 23, 2011.

Centers for Disease Control and Prevention. *Central line-associated bloodstream infection (CLABSI) Event.* Centers for Disease Control and Prevention. 2010. Available at: http://www.cdc.gov/nhsn/PDFs/pscManual/4PSC_CLABScurrent.pdf. Accessed December 23, 2011.

Centers for Disease Control and Prevention. *Emergency preparedness and response.* Centers for Disease Control and Prevention. 2012. Available at: http://www.bt.cdc.gov/. Accessed December 23, 2011.

Centers for Disease Control and Prevention. *National Healthcare Safety Network (NHSN).* Centers for Disease Control and Prevention. 2011. Available at: http://www.cdc.gov/nhsn/. Accessed December 27, 2011.

Centers for Disease Control and Prevention. *Surgical site infection (SSI) event.* Centers for Disease Control and Prevention. 2010. Available at: http://www.cdc.gov/nhsn/PDFs/pscManual/9pscSSIcurrent.pdf. Accessed December 23, 2011.

O'Grady NP, Alexander M, Burns LA, et al. *Guidelines for the prevention of intravascular catheter-related infections, 2011.* Centers for Disease Control and Prevention. 2011. Available at: http://www.cdc.gov/hicpac/pdf/guidelines/bsi-guidelines-2011.pdf. Accessed December 23, 2011.

Siegel JD, Rhinehart E, Jackson M, et al. Healthcare Infection Control Practices Advisory Committee Management of multidrug-resistant organisms in health care settings, 2006. *Am J Infect Control* 2007;35(10):S165–S193.

Verani JR, McGee L, Schrag SJ. *Prevention of perinatal group B streptococcal disease.* Centers for Disease Control and Prevention. 2010. Available at: http://www.cdc.gov/mmwr/preview/mmwrhtml/rr5910a1.htm?s_cid=rr5910a1_w. Accessed December 23, 2011.

Chapter 3

Blood Cultures

Clemence Cherson, MPA, CIC, CLS(ASCP)

Hospitalizations for sepsis have more than doubled in the United States between the years 2000 and 2008 according to a recent report released by the CDC's National Center for Health Statistics.[1] Data from the National Hospital Discharge Survey, 2008 shows a dramatic increase in the number of sepsis cases from 326,000 in 2000 to 727,000 in 2008. As the U.S. population has aged, increased use of invasive devices, extended device dwell time, increased antimicrobial use, and emerging antimicrobial resistance have all contributed to rising numbers of sepsis cases. Due to the high morbidity and mortality associated with septicemia, prompt and accurate diagnosis is essential. The laboratory test that is used to detect the presence of microorganisms in the blood is the blood culture.

Bacteremia types

According to the *Manual for Clinical Microbiology*, there are several types of bacteremia, depending on the source from which bacteria enters the bloodstream. Primary bacteremia refers to the presence of bacteria in the blood in the absence of an identifiable source or as the result of "silent" subclinical passage of bacteria from normally colonized sites in the body. This commonly occurs after dental procedures with no clinically significant sequelae. Secondary bacteremia refers to bacteria that enter the bloodstream from a primary site such as the lungs or a remote wound infection. Intermittent bacteremia occurs when bacteria are present in the blood for periods of time followed by nonbacteremic episodes. Continuous bacteremia occurs when patients with intravascular sites of infection such as endocarditis experience continuous seeding of the blood from a remote site. Many of these patients have very low quantities of bacteria in their blood, in spite of severe clinical symptoms.[2]

Primary and secondary bacteremia can result in sepsis, septic shock, or severe sepsis. Symptoms such as fever, chills, and tachycardia indicate sepsis, and the presence of hypotension along with sepsis indicates septic shock. Acute organ dysfunction, secondary to severe sepsis, has a 20 to 40 percent mortality rate. Because of the high morbidity and mortality associated with any type of sepsis, blood cultures have become the focal point of the sepsis workup and are critical to prompt diagnosis and treatment.[2]

The *Manual for Clinical Microbiology* defines infective endocarditis (IE) as "an infection of the lining of the heart chambers and valves. IE occurs when bacteremia or fungemia delivers infectious organisms to the surface of one or more heart valves where they adhere and eventually invade the valvular leaflets."[3] As with sepsis, blood culture results are vital to the diagnosis and management of patients with IE. Current culture techniques allow positive blood cultures to be obtained in more than 90 percent of infective endocarditis cases.[4] Continuous bacteremia is often the result of IE and, because of this, the timing of specimen collection for blood cultures is less important. Clinical and Laboratory Standards Institute recommends that blood cultures be collected 30 minutes prior to starting empiric antimicrobial therapy.[2]

The role of blood cultures in infection prevention and surveillance

With the advent of public reporting of healthcare-associated infections (HAIs) in many states and the recent CMS reporting requirements linked to Medicare reimbursement, there is significant interest in the collection and interpretation of blood cultures for confirmation of central venous catheter (often called *central lines*) infection.

Central Line–Related Blood Stream Infection (CRBSI) versus Central Line–Associated Blood Stream Infection (CLABSI)

CRBSI and CLABSI are often used interchangeably to describe bloodstream infections linked to intravascular catheters. However, it is important that clinicians and infection preventionists understand differences between the definitions of CRBSI and CLABSI to avoid misclassification.[2]

CRBSI

CRBSI is a rigorous clinical definition that requires specific laboratory testing to identify a catheter as the source of the BSI. The CRBSI definition is not used for surveillance, but rather for clinical research or determining diagnosis and treatment.[2]

To determine that an infection is directly related to the presence of the vascular access catheter, specific diagnostic criteria must be met. These criteria include one the following diagnostic tests:

- A positive semiquantitative (>15 colony-forming units [CFU/catheter segment]) or quantitative (>10^3 CFU/catheter segment) cultures in which the same organism (species and antibiogram) is isolated from the catheter segment and peripheral blood. Semiquantitative testing is the most commonly performed test due to its lower cost and simple technique. However, it does not detect organisms on the intraluminal surface of the catheter and may lead to a false-negative result, because bacterial biofilms may be present on both the exterior and/or interior surfaces of the device.[5]
- Simultaneous quantitative blood cultures with a ≥5:1 ratio central venous catheter (CVC) versus peripheral. This is the most reliable method but may not be available in all laboratories.
- Differential time-to-positivity between two blood cultures. If the blood culture obtained from the device is positive at least two hours before the percutaneously obtained culture, the infection is then related to the catheter.

A drawback in CRBSI testing is that the catheter must be removed. This can be problematic for the patient who requires venous access and increases the costs of care. Furthermore, the advantages and disadvantages of CRBSI remain controversial—large randomized controlled studies have not been conducted. As a result, the impact of prior antimicrobial therapy, the use of antimicrobial impregnated or coated catheters, the presence of multilumen catheters, and questions regarding the appropriate threshold for positive results complicate CRBSI analysis.[6]

CLABSI

CLABSI is a less scientifically rigorous definition and is only used for surveillance purposes. National Healthcare Safety Network (NHSN) defines CLABSI as a bloodstream infection that develops within 48 hours of insertion of a central venous or umbilical catheter. In the NHSN system, the infection must be described as primary or secondary during the reporting process. A primary CLABSI is (a) laboratory confirmed infection and (b) not an HAI meeting CDC/NHSN criteria for another body site.

Only lumened devices that terminate at or adjacent to the heart are included in CLABSI reporting. Pacemaker wires, extracorporeal membrane oxygenation (ECMO), intraaortic balloon pumps (IABPs), and femoral arterial catheters are not included as central catheters. However, peripherally inserted central catheters (PICCs) are part of CLABSI reporting in NHSN.

NHSN requires that, in addition to patient identification and demographic information, the following elements are reported:

- If the CLABSI has been detected after any procedure, and if so, when and what type
- If the CLABSI is part of the organization's in-plan MDRO/CDI reporting

- Risk factors identified
- Event details describing patient signs and symptoms
- Event details by laboratory findings (recognized pathogen from one of more cultures or common commensals from at least two or more cultures)
- Identified pathogens and their sensitivities

The culture of the catheter tip or any segment of the catheter is not a criterion for CLABSI.[7]

As value-based purchasing (VBP) becomes the norm in healthcare, the differences in CRBSI and CLABSI definitions, as well as their correct application, will become increasingly important. Currently, CMS requires that the CDC NHSN definition of CLABSI be used when reporting catheter-associated bloodstream infections for Medicare reimbursement. It is important to note that these surveillance definitions were not intended to be used for reimbursement purposes. The initial and ongoing intent of the CDC has been to develop a baseline reporting tool capable of producing comparable data across institutions and settings.

Blood Culture Tests

The accuracy of a blood culture can be impacted by a wide variety of factors, many of which pertain to skin antisepsis and/or specimen collection techniques.

Skin Antisepsis: In order to minimize the risk of contamination of the blood specimen with common commensals, the venipuncture site should be cleaned with an antiseptic. The most common antiseptics used are rubbing alcohol, tincture of iodine, povidone-iodine, iodophors, and chlorhexidine gluconate (CHG).

- Studies suggest that tincture of iodine and CHG are superior to povidone-iodine.
- It is important to follow the manufacturer's guidelines regarding the amount of time required for the antiseptic product to dry. If venipuncture is performed before the product has been in place long enough to achieve its full bactericidal effect, the integrity of the blood specimen may be jeopardized.
- CHG products are increasingly used as they are effective, require only 30 seconds to dry, and are not commonly associated with allergic reactions. CHG products do not need to removed or rinsed from the skin following venipuncture.
- Special considerations in pediatrics: CHG products are not approved for use with infants younger than 2 months of age. In addition, iodine-containing compounds should not be used with neonates due to the potential of developing subclinical hypothyroidism. For patients younger than 2 months of age, 70 percent isopropyl alcohol is an acceptable alternative.[8]

Specimen Collection: In order to assure the integrity of the specimen and the accuracy of testing, the following general guidelines for specimen collection must be followed:

- The volume of blood obtained for culture is a critical variable in detecting bacteremia or fungemia.
- Specimen collection from the central catheter is not recommended due to the possibility of intraluminal bacterial contamination of the device. Percutaneous venipuncture from two separate sites is preferred. Inguinal blood vessels (groin) should be avoided when other venipuncture sites are available.
- Follow institutional policy regarding any amount to be discarded when blood is sampled from indwelling vascular access devices.
- Blood specimens are only obtained from peripheral vascular access catheters at the time of insertion. If a patient has a peripheral catheter in place, the sample must be obtained percutaneously.
- It is critical that blood cultures be drawn prior to initiation of antibiotic therapy. Blood may not become sterile immediately following antimicrobial therapy. If empiric antibiotic therapy is initiated on an emergency basis, cultures should be obtained as soon as possible following the first dose.
- Single blood cultures should never be drawn from adult patients, as these results can be misleading.

- Only designated blood culture bottles are used for specimen collection. If blood is drawn into tubes, sodium polyanetholesulfonate (SPS) anticoagulant can inhibit microbial growth.
- The accidental contamination of blood culture bottles is unfortunately a common problem. It is essential that the tops, into which the blood specimen is transferred, remain sterile until the transfer is completed.
- For neonates and pediatric patients the volume of blood should be no more than 1 percent of the patient's total blood volume.[8]
- Blood culture bottles must be labeled following laboratory policy and should indicate not only the patient's name and other required identification information, but also the date, time, and location of specimen collection. If blood is obtained from a multilumen catheter, the specific lumen sampled should be described.
- Follow institutional policy regarding the removal of needleless connectors attached to the end of a central catheter. Although some products are labeled for blood sampling, many institutions require their removal to eliminate of the risk of contamination by biofilm that can accumulate in the interior components of these devices. The previously used connector is then discarded and a new, sterile connector is attached after the blood specimen is obtained.

See Table 3-1 for general guidelines for the collection of blood culture specimens.

Table 3-1: General Guidelines for Blood Culture Specimen Collection

Laboratory Test	Indications	Specific Microbes	Specimen Collection	Media	Time to Results	Test Type	Common Skin Contaminants	Interpretation
Routine blood cultures	Acute febrile episode	Aerobic and anaerobic Gram-positive cocci (e.g., *Streptococcus*, *Staphylococcus*), Gram-positive rods (*Bacillus*), Gram-negative rods (e.g., *Escherichia coli*, *Pseudomonas*), Gram-negative cocci (e.g., *Neisseria*)	• Collect two to three sets in a 24-hour period • Collect 20 mL per set divided into aerobic and anaerobic bottles	• Broth media is commonly used • All broth media contain anticoagulants to inhibit blood clot formation; SPS is the most common one used • Heparin, EDTA, and citrate are toxic to microorganisms; blood should not be collected in tubes containing these anticoagulants • Resins or proprietary activated charcoal are added to broth media formulations in order to remove antimicrobial agents from the blood	Incubated for 5 days	• Continuous monitoring systems incubate, agitate, and continuously monitor blood culture bottles for organism growth • The most common systems rely on increased CO_2 production by actively metabolizing organisms in the blood culture (BLC) bottles • A sensor at the bottom of the bottle will undergo acidification and either a colorimetric, fluorometric, or pressure change will occur that is detected by the system • Bottles are monitored every 10 minutes for changes in sensor; agitation is continuous to increase yields and improve time to recovery of organisms	• *Staphylococcus epidermidis*, *Bacillus* spp., *Propionibacterium*, *Streptococcus viridans* • In general, single cultures positive for these bacteria represent contamination • Multiple, separate cultures drawn from different sites growing one of these organisms are considered positive • Contamination rates of less than 3 percent are desired	• One positive bottle out of two bottles drawn is a positive result • BLC results are typically reported according to the organism's Gram stain reaction (positive or negative) and morphology seen on the slide (e.g., staphylococci are reported as Gram-positive cocci in clusters, enterococci are reported as Gram-positive cocci in chains and pairs, *E. coli* is Gram-negative and appears in rods)
Pediatric blood cultures	Suspected sepsis	As for adult patients; that is, aerobic and anaerobic Gram-positive cocci (e.g., *Streptococcus*, *Staphylococcus*), Gram-positive rods (*Bacillus*), Gram-negative rods (e.g., *Escherichia coli*, *Pseudomonas*), Gram-negative cocci (e.g., *Neisseria*)	• Collect two to three sets in a 24-hour period • For neonates and pediatric patients the volume of blood should be no more than 1 percent of the patient's total blood volume	Routine aerobic broth media	Five days	Pediatric bottles for continuous monitoring systems are available in order to accommodate smaller blood volumes	• As for adult patients; that is, *S. epidermidis*, *Bacillus* spp., *Propionibacterium*, *S. viridans* • In general, single cultures positive for these bacteria represent contamination • Multiple, separate cultures drawn from different sites growing one of these organisms are considered positive • Contamination rates of less than 3 percent are desired	• As for adult patients; that is, one positive bottle out of two bottles drawn is a positive result • BLC results are typically reported according to the organism's Gram stain reaction (positive or negative) and morphology seen on the slide (e.g., staphylococci are reported as Gram-positive cocci in clusters, enterococci are reported as Gram-positive cocci in chains and pairs, *E. coli* is Gram-negative and appears in rods)

Table 3-1: General Guidelines for Blood Culture Specimen Collection (*continued*)

Laboratory Test	Indications	Specific Microbes	Specimen Collection	Media	Time to Results	Test Type	Common Skin Contaminants	Interpretation
Blood cultures for rare and fastidious pathogens	Fever of unknown origin (FUO), IE, subacute endocarditis (SBE)	HACEK group (*Haemophilus* spp., *Actinobacillus* spp., *Cardiobacterium* spp., *Eikenella* spp., *Kingella* spp.), *Abiotrophia* spp., *Bartonella* spp., *Brucella* spp., *Campylobacter* spp., *Francisella* spp., *Helicobacter* spp., *Legionella* spp., *Leptospira* spp., *Mycoplasma* spp.	• Collect two to three sets in a 24-hour period • Collect 20 mL per set divided into aerobic and anaerobic bottles	No special media needed	Hold for 21 days if negative at 5 days	Continuous monitoring systems have demonstrated acceptable recovery of these organisms	• As for routine blood cultures; that is, *S. epidermidis, Bacillus* spp., *Propionibacterium, S. viridans* • In general, single cultures positive for these bacteria represent contamination • Multiple, separate cultures drawn from different sites growing one of these organisms are considered positive • Contamination rates of less than three percent are desired	• A phenomenon sometimes associated with these organisms is that of signal-positive (analyzer detects a positive signal from blood culture bottle)/Gram stain negative cultures; these organisms may have atypical morphology or unusually small size • In these cases clinical correlation should be attempted; culture may be held for 21 days
Mycobacterial blood cultures: Lysis centrifugation	When mycobacterial infections are suspected; not generally part of a sepsis workup	Growth of *Mycobacterium tuberculosis* as well as the nontuberculous mycobacteria	Consult laboratory	Optimal recovery requires supplementation of broth cultures with fatty acids (e.g., oleic acid), albumin, and carbon dioxide	Due to slow generation time, incubate minimum of 4 weeks	Automated broth-based media has shown superior recovery rates	As for routine blood cultures (see above)	Mycobacteria grow on solid or in broth media from the lysed material
Fungal blood cultures	When fungal infections are suspected	Generally yeast forms such as *Candida* and *Cryptococcus*	Consult laboratory	Recovery of yeasts is best in aerobic broth formulations Special media is not necessary	Five days for recovery of yeast	Continuous monitoring systems have demonstrated acceptable recovery rates of yeast	As for routine blood cultures (see above)	Yeast has a distinctive morphology on Gram stain and is reported as such

Table 3-1: General Guidelines for Blood Culture Specimen Collection (*continued*)

Laboratory Test	Indications	Specific Microbes	Specimen Collection	Media	Time to Results	Test Type	Common Skin Contaminants	Interpretation
Manual fungal blood culture systems	When fungal infections are suspected	Generally yeast forms such as *Candida* and *Cryptococcus*	Consult laboratory	Nutrient broth	Five days	Manual fungal blood culture—nutrient broth	• As for routine blood cultures; that is, *S. epidermidis*, *Bacillus* spp., *Propionibacterium*, *S. viridans* • In general, single cultures positive for these bacteria represent contamination • Multiple, separate cultures drawn from different sites growing one of these organisms are considered positive • Contamination rates of less than three percent are desired	Yeast has a distinctive morphology on Gram stain and is reported as such
	When fungal infections are suspected	Generally dimorphic forms such as *Histoplasma capsulatum* and filamentous fungi	Consult laboratory	Biphasic bottles (agar plus broth)	Four weeks' incubation required for reliable detection of dimorphic fungi	Biphasic fungal blood culture	As for routine blood cultures (see above)	Blood cultures for dimorphic fungi can only be grown by this method to recover both the yeast and the filamentous ("fuzzy") phases
	When fungal infections are suspected	Generally dimorphic forms such as *H. capsulatum* and filamentous fungi	Consult laboratory	• Fungal blood culture for dimorphic fungi • Yeast on one medium, "fuzzy," or filamentous on another medium at room temperature	Four weeks' incubation required for reliable detection of dimorphic fungi	Lysis centrifugation fungal blood culture	As for routine blood cultures (see above)	Blood cultures for dimorphic fungi can only be grown by this method to recover both the yeast and the filamentous ("fuzzy") phases

Table 3-1: General Guidelines for Blood Culture Specimen Collection *(continued)*

Laboratory Test	Indications	Specific Microbes	Specimen Collection	Media	Time to Results	Test Type	Common Skin Contaminants	Interpretation
Parasite blood cultures	When parasitic blood infections are suspected	Only a few parasites can be cultured: *Entamoeba histolytica*, *Naegleria fowleri*, *Acanthamoeba* spp., *Trichomonas vaginalis*, *Trypanosoma cruzi*, and *Leishmania*	Consult laboratory	Consult laboratory	Consult laboratory	Blood culture—rule out parasites	• As for routine blood cultures; that is, *S. epidermidis*, *Bacillus* spp., *Propionibacterium*, *S. viridans* • In general, single cultures positive for these bacteria represent contamination • Multiple, separate cultures drawn from different sites growing one of these organisms are considered positive • Contamination rates of less than three percent are desired	
Viral blood cultures	Suspected acute phase of a viral infection	Adenovirus, cytomegalovirus, herpes simplex, influenza, varicella-zoster	Laboratory specific; consult with laboratory	Growth on monolayer cell cultures	Consult laboratory	• Continuous monitoring systems cannot identify the presence of virus particles in blood • Use viral polymerase chain reaction (PCR) testing in the blood	As for routine blood cultures (see above)	
Viral blood culture: Nucleic acid testing	Suspected acute phase of a viral infection	Common viruses such as HIV, enteroviruses, hepatitis C, human papillomaviruses, varicella-zoster viruses	Consult with laboratory	By PCR testing	Consult laboratory	Viral PCR blood test	As for routine blood cultures (see above)	Test detects viral DNA or rNA present in the sample

References

1. Hall MJ, Williams SN, DeFrances CJ, Golosinskiy A. *Inpatient care for septicemia or sepsis: A challenge for patients and hospitals.* NCHS data brief, no. 62. Hyattsville, MD: National Center for Health Statistics. 2011. Available at: http://www.cdc.gov/nchs/data/databriefs/db62.pdf. Accessed April 16, 2012.

2. Clinical and Laboratory Standards Institute (CLSI). *Principles and Procedures for Blood Cultures: Approved Guideline.* CLSI document M47-A. Wayne, PA: Clinical and Laboratory Standards Institute, 2007.

3. Miller JM, Krisher K, Holmes HT. General Principles of Specimen Collection and Handling. In: Murray PR, Baron EJ, Jorgensen H, Landry ML, Pfaller MA, eds. *Manual of Clinical Microbiology*, 9th ed. Washington, DC: ASM, 2007.

4. Brusch JL, Cunha BA. *Infective Endocarditis.* Medscape Reference. 2011. Available at: http://emedicine.medscape.com\article\216650-overview. Accessed May 20, 2011.

5. Ryder MA. Catheter-Related Infections: It's All About Biolfim. Topics in Advanced Practice Nursing eJournal.2005;5(3). Available at: http://www.medscape.com/viewarticle/508109. Accessed April 11, 2012.

6. Raad I, Kassar R, Ghannam D, Chaftari AM, Hachem R, Jiang Y. Management of the catheter in documented catheter-related coagulase-negative staphylococcal bacteremia: remove or retain? *Clin Infect Dis.* 2009;49(8):1187–1194.

7. Centers for Disease Control and Prevention. National Healthcare Safety Network (NHSN). CDC. 2012. Available at www.cdc.gov/nhsn. Accessed April 11, 2012.

8. Murphy C, Andrus M, Barnes S, et al. *Guide to the Elimination of Catheter-Related Bloodstream Infections.* Washington, DC: APIC, 2009.

Chapter 4

Microbial Immunology

Kathy Aureden, MS, MT(ASCP)SI, CIC

Antigens are cellular components or molecules that are recognized as foreign and "nonself" by the body, including those that are introduced during a communicable disease exposure or when a person is vaccinated. The immune response triggered by the presence of the antigen(s) results in production of molecules called antibodies that aid in the elimination of the foreign "invader." Laboratory tests to detect antigen or antibody are called serologic tests. Serologic tests that detect pathogen-specific antigens or antibodies are often used in the diagnosis of communicable diseases, or to verify immunity to disease. The infection preventionist can make use of these tests in surveillance for communicable disease and for the determination of the immune status of a patient or healthcare worker to a given communicable or vaccine preventable disease. Hepatitis B virus testing serves as a good example of the use of serologic tests in communicable disease detection as well as immune status verification. The panel of hepatitis B virus tests commonly ordered includes tests that detect hepatitis B virus *antigens* (e.g., HBsAg) and tests that detect hepatitis B virus specific *antibodies* (e.g., HBsAb) as well as other markers. The reader is directed to Weinbaum et al. (2011) for a comprehensive algorithm and interpretations of the various hepatitis B virus serologic tests.

Serologic Tests for Antibodies

Serologic tests for immune responses to a specific pathogen are reported in terms of total antibodies (all classes of immunoglobulins), or as a specific immunoglobulin (Ig) class of antibody (e.g., IgG, IgM). The immunoglobulin class of an antibody is helpful in determining if antibodies are present due to *acute* disease, or if the antibodies are detected because the patient is in the *convalescent* stage, or has *immune* memory of a prior exposure to a specific disease-causing pathogen.

During the primary immune response after communicable disease pathogen or vaccine is encountered, the class of antibody that is produced first is IgM. IgG antibodies develop a few weeks later and are a good indication of the convalescence period and generally mark the establishment of long-term immunity to the pathogen. The IgG antibody *titer* is the quantitative measure of antibody. An IgG-specific antibody titer may remain detectable for months, years, or for life. IgM antibodies to the specific pathogen wane over time and will become undetectable as the IgG antibody titer rises. The class of immunoglobulin called IgA is the predominant antibody of secretions but may also be present in serum and may occasionally be included in testing for some infectious diseases (Turgeon, 2009).

When exposure to a pathogen occurs again after a primary exposure, or after a booster vaccination, a secondary or "anamnestic" immune response occurs. The characteristics of the immunoglobulin class response, magnitude of antibody titers, and the antibody response timing differs during a secondary immune response from a primary response (see Figure 1). During a secondary response, the immune response is boosted and will occur faster and stronger. The secondary immune response to a communicable disease exposure often prevents the development of disease during a subsequent exposure, or will result in an infection that is milder and quickly self-limiting.

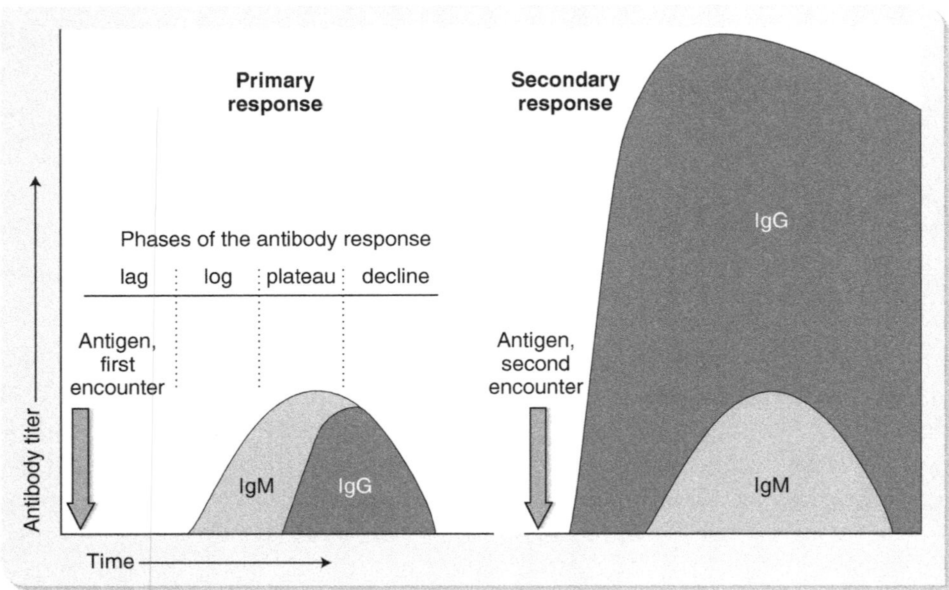

Figure 4-1: Primary and secondary antibody responses.

From: Doan T, Melvold R, Waltenbaugh C. *Concise Medical Immunology.* Baltimore: Lippincott Williams & Wilkins, 2005

As shown in the Figure 4-1, detection of IgM alone is typical of early, active (acute) infection. IgM and IgG antibodies may both be detectable in the plateau phase of a primary immune response. In general, high titers of IgG detected at the same time as very low (or not detectable) IgM titers indicates immunity and is associated with convalescence, booster response, or past infection.

Laboratory methodologies used to identify and quantify specific antibodies include enzyme-linked immunoassays (EIAs), fluorescent assays (FAs), immunodiffusion, Western blot, hemagglutination, latex agglutination, and others. Results may be quantified as titers or units, or resulted semiquantitatively as positive/negative, detected/not detected, or present/not present.

Serologic Tests for Antigens

Laboratory tests that detect specific bacterial, viral, cellular, or proteinaceous antigens often use antibodies specific to the antigen of interest. In some laboratory methodologies, the antibody used to detect antigen is tagged with a detectable molecule. In others, a tagged antigen-antibody "sandwich" is used to detect the antigen of interest. Examples of these assays include EIAs, immunofluorescent immunoassays, histochemical stain tests, chemiluminescent assays, immunodiffusion assays, and different types of electrophoresis assays. In addition, there are assays that use polymerase chain reaction (PCR), genetic probes, and other specialized gene-based methodologies, such as DNA or RNA viral load tests, to detect specific antigens.

Some testing methodologies will be reported as a qualitative result, indicating that the antigen/antibody is present or not. An example of this type of qualitative reporting is the total hepatitis A antibody test that is reported as "detected." Otherwise, the result will be quantitative, indicating how much is present. For example, an HIV RNA viral load is reported as "x" number of copies.

A panel of tests for some infectious diseases may contain both antigen and antibody test results. The panel of tests for the diagnosis of hepatitis B (including antigen and antibody detection) provides a good example, as demonstrated below in Figure 4-2.

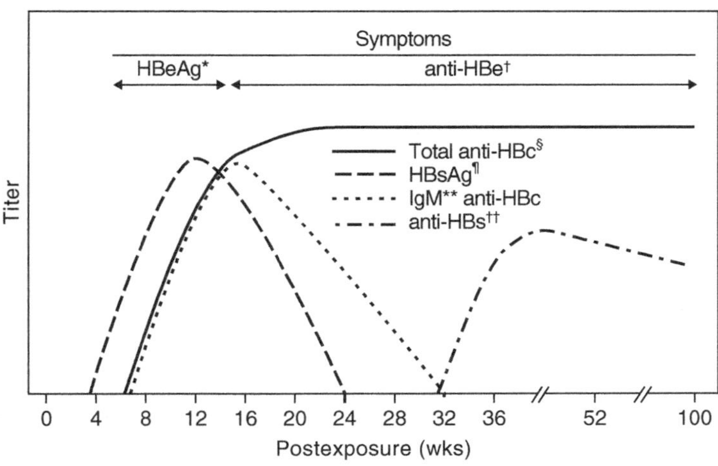

* Hepatitis B e antigen.
† Antibody to HBeAg.
§ Antibody to hepatitis B core antigen.
¶ Hepatitis B surface antigen.
** Immunoglobulin M.
†† Antibody to HBsAg.

Figure 4-2: Acute hepatitis B virus infection and recovery.

From: Weinbaum CM, Williams I, Mast EE, Wang SA, Finelli L, Wasley A et al. Recommendations for Identification and Public Health Management of Persons with Chronic Hepatitis B Virus Infection. *MMWR* 2008; 57(RR-8): 1–10. Available at http://www.cdc.gov/mmwr/pdf/rr/rr5708.pdf. Accessed August 1, 2011.

Table 4-1: Overview of Serologic Tests

Lab Test	Indications	Specific Microbe/Disease	Specimen	Frequency	Test Type	Interpretation	Advantages/Disadvantages	Key Points
Immune Response Testing								
Total antibody, pathogen specific	• Acute and convalescent stage of infectious disease in question • Immunity	Bacterial, viral, fungal, spirochete, parasite	Serum, spinal fluid, other body fluids (rare)	Test of immunity	• EIA • Chromogenic immunoassay • Hemagglutination (HA)/HA inhibition • Latex agglutination • Fluorescent antibody tests • Western blot	Presence of total pathogen-specific antibodies indicates past or current immune response	Cannot distinguish between current and past infection	Best used as verification of past immune response with subsequent immunity
IgM antibody, pathogen specific	Developing (active) or current infection	Bacterial, viral, fungal, spirochete, parasite	Serum, spinal fluid, other body fluids (rare)	IgM present in *acute specimen* and not present in *convalescent specimen* obtained 4 weeks after acute specimen	• EIA • Chromogenic immunoassay • HA/HA inhibition • Latex agglutination • Fluorescent antibody tests • Western blot	Indicates acute immune response	• IgM antibody levels drop to undetectable levels within a few weeks of immune response • Exact timing of undetectable IgM varies per pathogen and per type of test assay	• In acute phase of illness, IgM antibodies are detected • In convalescent phase, IgG antibodies are detected
IgG antibody, pathogen specific	Recent or past infection	Bacterial, viral, fungal, spirochete, parasite	Serum, spinal fluid, other body fluids (rare)	Not present in *acute specimen* but present in *convalescent specimen* obtained 4 weeks after acute specimen	• EIA • Chromogenic immunoassay • HA/HA inhibition • Latex agglutination • Fluorescent antibody tests • Western blot	Indicates convalescence or past immunity	Rising versus falling versus maintenance IgG titers (levels) cannot be determined without sequential testing	"Seroconversion" of antibody test loosely defined as fourfold rise in IgG antibody titer between acute and convalescent specimen
IgA antibody, pathogen specific	Immune response elicited in secretions	Pathogens of respiratory tract or gut	• Serum • Spinal fluid, saliva, other body fluids (rarely tested)	N/A	• EIA • HA/HA inhibition • Latex agglutination • Fluorescent antibody tests • Western blot	For selected infectious diseases, may indicate acute immune response	Indicated for specific infectious diseases only	• Some diagnostic value in testing for congenital toxoplasmosis • *Helicobacter* infection • Herpes simplex infection
Pathogen-specific DNA, RNA, or antigen testing								
	Presence of pathogen-specific genetic material or cellular antigens	Bacterial, viral, fungal	Serum, spinal fluid, saliva, other body fluids	During acute illness	• Molecular test assays (e.g., PCR) • EIA • HA/HA inhibition • Latex agglutination • Fluorescent antibody tests • T cell proliferation assays • Electrophoresis	Detectable when pathogen is present in specimen	Presence of cellular elements may clinically correlate with acute disease, although does not differentiate between live and dead	• Assay specificity and sensitivity varies in populations with and without disease • Requires clinical correlation

Table 4-1: Overview of Serologic Tests (continued)

Lab Test	Indications	Specific Microbe/Disease	Specimen	Frequency	Test Type	Interpretation	Advantages/Disadvantages	Key Points
Selected Pathogens								
Hepatitis C total antibody	Test of exposure and immunity to hepatitis C virus (HCV)	HCV infection or immunization	Serum	Test of immunity	EIA	Immunity to HCV	Cannot distinguish between current and past infection	Verifies HCV infection and immunity current or past
Hepatitis C IgM antibody	Test of exposure and developing immunity to HCV (acute phase)	HCV infection or immunization	Serum	During acute illness	EIA	Current HCV infection	Detectable during acute illness, false positives are possible	Detectable in acute phase of HCV infection
Hepatitis C IgG antibody	Test of exposure and immunity to HCV (convalescent phase)	HCV infection or immunization	Serum	If acute illness, repeat in 4 weeks (convalescent specimen)	EIA	Recent or past HCV infection	Interpretation depends on phase of illness (acute, convalescent, past)	Detectable in convalescent phase of HCV infection
HCV viral load, HCV RNA titers	Test for acute or chronic HCV	Acute infection or chronic HCV disease	Serum	Periodic tests can be done to evaluate therapeutic response	Molecular tests (e.g., DNA or RNA PCR)	• Confirmation of disease in patients with indeterminate results of HCV antibody results or in immunosuppressed patients • Test of therapeutic response	• Not routine in many hospital labs • Usually available at reference laboratories	• Earliest detectable marker for acute disease • Quantitative results • Good specificity and sensitivity for disease resolution
Note: Hepatitis B virus (HBV): accurate interpretation requires an array of tests (e.g., hepatitis B panels for acute infection, chronic infection, or immunization)								
Hepatitis B surface antibody (HBsAb)	Test of exposure and immunity to hepatitis B	HBV infection or immunization	Serum	Test of immunity (see Figure 2)	EIA	Immunity to HBV (after infection or HBV immunization)		Indication of immunity to HBV
Hepatitis B core IgM antibody (HBcAb-IgM)	Test of HBV and developing immunity	HBV infection	Serum	During acute illness	• EIA • Others	Indication of developing immunity: detectable during early stages of acute disease		Not elicited by HBV immunization
Hepatitis B core total antibody (HBcAb-total)	Test of exposure and immunity during HBV	HBV infection	Serum	Test of immunity (see Figure 2)	• EIA • Others	Indication of developing or established immunity (HBcIgM declines but HBcIgG remains detectable)		Not elicited by HBV immunization
Hepatitis B surface antigen (HBsAg)	Test for acute HBV	HBV infection or immunization	Serum	During acute illness or carrier state (see Figure 2)	• EIA • Others	• Detectable during incubation period of acute disease • Not detectable during disease convalescence and resolution	Patients are contagious when they are positive antigen (HBsAg) and negative for antibody (HBsAB)	Immunity: HBsAg will be undetectable when HBsAb is present after infection or immunization

Table 4-1: Overview of Serologic Tests *(continued)*

Lab Test	Indications	Specific Microbe/Disease	Specimen	Frequency	Test Type	Interpretation	Advantages/Disadvantages	Key Points
Hepatitis Be antigen	Test of HBV disease	HBV infection	Serum	During acute illness or carrier state (see Figure 2)	• EIA • Others	• Detectable during incubation period of acute disease • Not detectable during disease convalescence and resolution	• One indicator of carrier state for HBV • Important supplemental test in pregnant women at risk of HBV disease	Not elicited by HBV immunization
Hepatitis antibody	Early immune response to HBV	HBV infection	Serum	Test of immunity (see Figure 2)	• EIA • Others	Earliest indication of developing immunity to HBV after infection		Not elicited by HBV immunization
Hepatitis delta (hepatitis D) antibody	Hepatitis D primary infection or coinfection with HBV	Acute infection or coinfection in chronic HBsAg positive carrier	Serum	N/A	• EIA, PCR, RIA • Tissue staining (virus particles in liver)	Important prognostic tool in chronic HBV carrier (HBsAg positive) at risk of coinfection with hepatitis delta	• Not routine in many hospital labs • Usually available at reference laboratories	Important to identify apparently healthy HBV carriers at risk of serious liver damage due to coinfection
HBV DNA viral load, HBV RNA probe		Acute infection or chronic HBV disease	Serum	Periodic testing used to evaluate therapeutic response	Molecular tests (e.g., DNA or RNA PCR)	• Confirmation of disease in patients with indeterminate results of HBV panel • Test of therapeutic response	• Not routine in many hospital labs • Usually available at reference laboratories	• Quantitative results • Good specificity and sensitivity for disease resolution
HIV-1 and HIV-2 antibody tests; HIV p24 antibody tests	HIV or AIDS	Human immunodeficiency viruses	Serum, blood, plasma, saliva	• Test of HIV infection • Test for seroconversion during 6 months after exposure	• EIA (including waived rapid tests) and confirmatory Western blot/immunoblot • IFA • Line immunoassay	HIV antibodies present in HIV and AIDS	Known false positive and false negative EIA tests	Positive EIA tests to be confirmed by Western blot or immunoblot assay
HIV antigen detection and viral load	HIV or AIDS	Human immunodeficiency viruses	Serum, cerebrospinal fluid	May be detectable 4 to 6 weeks after exposure	• EIA for p24 antigen • PCR for HIV-1	• Active infection • Therapeutic response monitoring	• Sensitivity of EIA is poor • PCR for HIV-1 is very sensitive	May be positive before seroconversion per HIV antibody tests
Lyme/borreliosis antibody testing	Lyme disease	*Borrelia burgdorferi* (spirochete)	Serum, joint fluid	Acute and convalescent specimens (obtained about 4 weeks apart)	• Enzyme linked immunosorbent assay (ELISA) and EIA • Confirmatory Western blot is recommended • PCR molecular testing of joint fluid	• IgM antibodies in acute specimen, IgG antibodies in convalescent specimen • For Western blot, see test notes for specific "bands" present in Lyme disease	• EIA and ELISA tests may have low specificity and sensitivity • Western blot results (bands) have varying cross-reactivity with antibodies to other non-Lyme spirochetes	• EIA and ELISA tests should be confirmed by Western blot and/or PCR tests • PCR tests of joint fluid are specific but may not be very sensitive

Table 4-1: Overview of Serologic Tests *(continued)*

Lab Test	Indications	Specific Microbe/ Disease	Specimen	Frequency	Test Type	Interpretation	Advantages/ Disadvantages	Key Points
Legionella pneumophila antibody tests	Legionnaire's disease, legionellosis, Pontiac fever	Legionnaire's disease, legionellosis		Acute and convalescent specimens (obtained about 4 weeks apart)	• Western blot • EIA • Fluorescent antibody test	Fourfold rise in titer between acute and convalescent specimens, IgM antibodies present only during acute phase	Good sensitivity and specificity if results of paired (acute and convalescent) are done	Legionella serotype 1 is most common clinical isolate; however, others are possible in human disease
Legionella pneumophila urinary antigen tests	Legionnaire's disease, legionellosis, Pontiac fever	Legionnaire's disease, legionellosis	Urine		• Chromogenic immunoassay • EIA • Fluorescent antibody test	During acute illness, test of choice is urine antigen test	Good sensitivity and nearly 100% specificity	Environmental testing for *Legionella* in water systems is important in outbreak investigations
Respiratory syncytial virus (RSV) antigen test	RSV infection in young children and immunocompromised patients	RSV	Nasopharyngeal specimen	Acute illness	• EIA and other immunoassays • PCR	Diagnostic aid during acute illness, test of choice is antigen test	• EIA rapid test has lower sensitivity than PCR • Nasal, pharyngeal, and tracheal specimens are *not* optimal for clinical testing	Antibody testing not useful for clinical management of acute illness
Influenza antigen test	Influenza-like illness testing	• Influenza A and influenza B • Check test manufacturer's information on which influenza A and B strains are detected	Nasal, nasopharyngeal, and pharyngeal specimens	During acute illness	• EIA and other immunoassays • PCR	Diagnostic aid during acute illness	• EIA "rapid" test has lower sensitivity than PCR • EIA rapid test differentiates between A and B strains • PCR further identifies strains (hemagglutinin-H and neuraminidase-N)	• Testing reliability higher during influenza-like illness season • PCR tests can validate strain type of influenza (e.g., H1N1, H3N2, etc.)
Influenza antibody tests	Proof of immunity	Influenza A and influenza B	Serum		• EIA and other immunoassays • PCR	Immune response to influenza A and influenza B		• Not useful in acute illness • Validates immunity (past infection, immunization)
Group A streptococcus antigen test	Pharyngitis	Beta hemolytic group A *Streptococcus pyogenes*	Pharyngeal specimens	During acute illness	• EIA rapid test • Immunochromogenic immunoassay	Positive in group A streptococcal pharyngitis	• Low sensitivity • Cannot differentiate live and dead bacteria • Recommend throat culture if clinically indicated	Waived laboratory test can be done in clinical settings (doctor's office, emergency department, etc.)

Table 4-1: Overview of Serologic Tests (*continued*)

Lab Test	Indications	Specific Microbe/Disease	Specimen	Frequency	Test Type	Interpretation	Advantages/Disadvantages	Key Points
Group A streptococcus antibodies	Rheumatic fever, post-streptococcal glomerulonephritis	Beta hemolytic group A *Streptococcus pyogenes*	Serum	Post-streptococcal infection	• EIA • IFA • Other antibody immunoassay	Immune response to group A streptococcus	Not useful in acute infections	Can aid in diagnosis of immune complication following group A streptococcus infection
Fungal infections (respiratory and systemic); antigen and antibody tests	Fungal infection: respiratory, disseminated (systemic)	*Histoplasma capsulatum*: Darling disease, Ohio river valley fever, etc.	• Serum for antibody tests • Tissue, blood, sputum, urine for antigen tests	Acute and convalescent specimens for antibody testing, clinical specimen as available for antigen testing	• Complement fixation • Immunodiffusion • PCR	Fourfold rise in titer between acute and convalescent specimens	• Variable specificity and sensitivity for antibody tests, urine antigen test may be more clinically useful in disseminated disease • Cross-reactivity with other fungi are possible with antibody testing	Supplementary to fungal culture
Fungal infections (respiratory and systemic); antigen and antibody tests	Fungal infection: respiratory, disseminated (systemic)	*Blastomyces dermatitidis*	Serum for antibody tests	Acute and convalescent specimens for antibody testing	• Complement fixation • Immunodiffusion		• Poor test reliability • Fungal culture and tissue stains are gold standard	Supplementary to fungal culture and tissue stains
Fungal infections (respiratory and systemic); antigen and antibody tests	Fungal infection: respiratory, disseminated (systemic)	*Coccidioides immitis*: desert fever, valley fever	• Serum for antibody tests • Clinical specimen (tissue, sputum, etc.)	Acute and convalescent specimens for antibody testing, clinical specimen as available for antigen testing	• Complement fixation • Immunodiffusion • Antigen identification by fluorescent antibody test on clinical specimen	Fourfold rise in titer between acute and convalescent specimens	• Poor test reliability • Fungal culture and tissue stains are gold standard	Supplementary to fungal culture and tissue stains
Cryptococcus antigen test; cryptococcus antibody test	Pulmonary disease or meningitis (brain disease)	*Cryptococcus neoformans*	Serum, cerebrospinal fluid		• Latex agglutination antigen test • Fluorescent antibody and complement fixation antibody tests	Presence of antigen indicative of disease	High titers in antigen tests generally reflect more serious disease	Decrease in antigen and increase in antibody indicates recovery
Antibody testing; vaccine-preventable childhood diseases	• Acute infection • Verification of immunity	Measles, mumps, rubella, chickenpox, pertussis	Serum	During acute illness, in convalescence, and as test of immunity	EIA for IgM- and IgG-specific antibodies	• IgM positive and IgG negative: acute disease or recent immunization • IgM and IgG positive: recent infection or false positive results • IgM negative and IgG positive: immunity due to past infection or immunization	• Aid in diagnosis of acute infection in neonates, children, adults • Verification of immunity in health-care workers during exposure situation	IgM antibody tests are used to aid in diagnosis of neonatal infection because maternal IgG may cross placenta and be present in neonatal blood specimen

Table 4-1: Overview of Serologic Tests *(continued)*

Lab Test	Indications	Specific Microbe/ Disease	Specimen	Frequency	Test Type	Interpretation	Advantages/ Disadvantages	Key Points
Antigen or molecular testing: measles virus	Active infection	Rubeola	Throat or nasopharyngeal swabs, urine specimens		PCR	When detected, may indicate active infection	Cannot differentiate active from inactive virus	Supplementary to viral culture
Antigen or molecular testing: mumps virus	Active infection	Paramyxovirus of the genus *Rubulavirus*	Oral or buccal swab specimen		PCR	When detected, may indicate active infection	Cannot differentiate active from inactive virus	Supplementary to viral culture
Antigen or molecular testing: chickenpox/varicella zoster virus	Active infection: primary chickenpox or zoster (shingles)		Vesicular lesions		PCR	When detected, may indicate active infection	Cannot differentiate active from inactive virus	Supplementary to viral culture
Pertussis (*Bordetella*)	Active infection	*Bordetella pertussis*	Nasopharyngeal swab specimen		PCR	When detected, may indicate active infection	Cannot differentiate live and dead bacteria	
Antigen testing for sexually transmitted diseases	Sexually transmitted diseases	*Chlamydia trachomatis* and *Neisseria gonorrhoeae*	Genital specimen		PCR	When detected, may indicate active infection		
Antigen testing for syphilis	Sexually transmitted diseases	*Treponema pallidum*	Serum		• Nonspecific treponemal antibody tests (e.g., RPR rapid reagin antibody, VDRL on cerebrospinal fluid, etc.) • Specific treponema specific antibody by IFA (FTA-ABS), hemagglutination (MHA-TP) • EIA recombinant wild type *T. pallidum*	Used to diagnose active infection (specific antibody tests) and to monitor therapeutic progress (semiquantitative nonspecific antibody tests)		Nonspecific treponemal antibody tests are used for screening but are confirmed by specific treponemal test
Norovirus	• Vomiting and diarrheal disease: acute infection • Outbreaks	Norwalk-like viruses (NLV) in *Caliciviridae* family	Stool and emesis specimens		PCR	Diagnosis of acute infection	For outbreak detection, test is offered by state health departments	• Lab testing most useful for investigating outbreaks • Clinical diagnosis often sufficient in this self-limiting disease

Table 4-1: Overview of Serologic Tests *(continued)*

Lab Test	Indications	Specific Microbe/ Disease	Specimen	Frequency	Test Type	Interpretation	Advantages/ Disadvantages	Key Points
Viral encephalitis and meningitis: antigen/molecular tests and antibody tests	Symptoms of brain disease during mosquito (vector) season	West Nile virus, Eastern Equine encephalitis, St. Louis encephalitis, La Crosse encephalitis, etc.	Serum, cerebrospinal fluid		• For antibodies: ELISA, fluorescent antibody test, complement fixation, hemagglutination, antibody neutralization • For virus: PCR or viral culture	• IgM positive and IgG negative: acute disease • IgM and IgG positive: recent infection or false positive results • IgM negative and IgG positive: immunity due to past infection	• Antibody detection generally not useful in diagnosis during acute phase of illness • Viral culture or PCR may be available	• Antibody detection verifies immune response • Antigen detection and viral culture are of diagnostic value during acute illness

References

Weinbaum CM, Williams I, Mast EE, Wang SA, Finelli L, Wasley A, et al. Recommendations for Identification and Public Health Management of Persons with Chronic Hepatitis B Virus Infection. *MMWR* 2008; 57(RR-8): 1–10. Available at http://www.cdc.gov/mmwr/pdf/rr/rr5708.pdf. Accessed August 1, 2011.

Turgeon, ML. *Immunology and Serology in Laboratory Medicine*. 4th ed. St. Louis: Mosby, 2009.

Doan T, Melvold R, Waltenbaugh C. *Concise Medical Immunology*, 1st ed. Baltimore: Lippincott Williams & Wilkins, 2005.

Todar K. Immune Defense against Microbial Pathogens. Kenneth Todar: *Todar's Online Textbook of Bacteriology*. 2005. http://textbookofbacteriology.net/immune.html. Accessed August 1, 2011.

Centers for Disease Control and Prevention. *Interpretation of Hepatitis B Serologic Test Results*. Centers for Disease Control and Prevention: Centers for Disease Control and Prevention. Available at http://www.cdc.gov/hepatitis/HBV/PDFs/SerologicChartv8.pdf. Accessed August 1, 2011.

Additional Resources

Conely J and Portugal F. *The Immunology Lab*. Howard Hughes Medical Institute: Biointeractive Virtual Lab. 2012. Available at http://www.hhmi.org/biointeractive/vlabs/index.html. Accessed August 1, 2011.

Centers for Disease Control and Prevention. *Shingles: Collecting Specimens for Varicella Zoster Virus (Chicken Pox & Shingles) Testing*. Centers for Disease Control and Prevention: Centers for Disease Control and Prevention. 2011 Available at http://www.cdc.gov/shingles/lab-testing/collecting-specimens.html. Accessed August 1, 2011.

Centers for Disease Control and Prevention. *Legionellosis Resource Site*. Centers for Disease Control and Prevention: Centers for Disease Control and Prevention. 2011. Available at http://www.cdc.gov/legionella/. Accessed August 1, 2011.

Centers for Disease Control and Prevention. *Mumps: Overview of Laboratory Confirmation by IgM Serology*. Centers for Disease Control and Prevention: Centers for Disease Control and Prevention. 2010. http://www.cdc.gov/mumps/lab/overview-serology.html. Accessed August 1, 2011.

Centers for Disease Control and Prevention. *Measles Serology*. Centers for Disease Control and Prevention: Centers for Disease Control and Prevention. 2009. Available at http://www.cdc.gov/measles/lab-tools/serology.html. Accessed August 15, 2011.

Centers for Disease Control and Prevention. *Respiratory Syncytial Virus Infection (RSV)*. Centers for Disease Control and Prevention: Centers for Disease Control and Prevention. 2010. http://www.cdc.gov/rsv/. Accessed August 10, 2011.

Chapter 5

Antimicrobial Testing

Carol Sykora, MT(ASCP), MEd, CIC

Clinical microbiology laboratories analyze organisms suspected of causing infectious processes in the patient. Once an infectious organism is identified, the lab performs susceptibility testing, using a variety of testing methods. Only if the organism is capable of exhibiting resistance to commonly used antimicrobials, or if its susceptibility cannot be predicted from its identity, is susceptibility testing performed. Not all identified organisms warrant susceptibility testing.

The American National Standards Institute (ANSI) has accredited the Clinical and Laboratory Standards Institute (CLSI), a voluntary, international, nonprofit organization, to develop standards and guidelines and provide interpretative education to the healthcare community in the United States.

The CLSI Subcommittee on Antimicrobial Susceptibility Testing establishes the test methods, interpretive criteria, and quality control parameters used in antimicrobial susceptibility testing. The CLSI interpretive susceptibility breakpoints are based on generic reference testing methods. Commercial devices commonly used for susceptibility testing (e.g., Phoenix, Vitek, Microscan, Aris) are regulated by the U.S. Food and Drug Administration (FDA) in the United States. Per the CLSI, "In the US, laboratories that use FDA-approved susceptibility testing devices are allowed to use the FDA interpretive breakpoints. Either FDA or CLSI susceptibility interpretive breakpoints are acceptable to clinical laboratory accrediting bodies. Policies in other countries may vary."

Table 5-1 lists the various methods of antimicrobial testing performed on nonfastidious aerobic organisms. In addition to the methods listed, there are confirmatory tests (e.g., D-test, modified Hodge test, etc.) that can be performed to detect resistance mechanisms of the organisms. Need for these confirmatory tests vary per the testing methodology and antibiotic breakpoints, and will not be described in this chapter.

Standardized methods for susceptibility testing are only available for a limited subset of organisms. For many organisms, there are no interpretive criteria available. Additional susceptibility testing can be performed on these isolated organisms, per physician request, but the results are not interpretable using known susceptibility criteria and therefore this testing is discouraged.

Clinical microbiologists use the Gram stain to help them identify bacteria. The Gram stain separates organisms into two groups known as Gram positives and Gram negatives according to their cell structure. Differences in the structures of these two groups account for the differences in their susceptibility to various antimicrobial agents.

Antimicrobial agents impact the growth of bacteria either by killing them (bactericidal) or impairing their ability to grow or multiply (bacteriostatic). These agents impact their bacterial targets through specific modes of action. They may:

- Interfere with cell wall synthesis
- Inhibit protein synthesis
- Interfere with nucleic acid synthesis
- Inhibit a metabolic pathway

Antimicrobial agents within the same class typically have the same modes of action.

Table 5-2 lists the classes of antimicrobial agents and their antibiotic activity.

In response to the antimicrobial agents used to kill or impair bacteria, bacteria have developed a number of ways to resist these agents and survive. Their resistance mechanisms include:

- Producing enzymes to destroy the antimicrobial agent before it reaches its target
- Modifying the agent so that it no longer interacts with its target
- Altering their cell wall makeup, making them impermeable to the antimicrobial agent
- Altering the bacterial cell target site so that the antimicrobial agent no longer binds to it
- Using an efflux pump that expels the antimicrobial agent from the bacteria before it can impact the bacteria
- Developing alternative metabolic pathways that bypass the reaction inhibited by the antimicrobial agent

Bacteria that have developed resistance to several classes of antimicrobial agents are categorized as multidrug-resistant organisms (MDRO). MDROs are increasingly isolated in more and more species of organisms. Infection preventionists (IPs) began recognizing the significance of MDROs with the development of resistant Gram-positive organisms, such as oxacillin-resistant *Staphylococcus aureus* and vancomycin-resistant *Enterococcus faecium* and *faecalis*. IPs were aware of the increasing resistance developing in the community-acquired infections due to infectious organisms such as *Neisseria gonorrhea* and *Mycobacterium tuberculosis*. We learned of resistance developing in strains of viral organisms, too, such as the human immunodeficiency virus (HIV). Most recently the microbiology community has been alerting IPs to the multidrug-resistance identified in Gram-negative organisms such as *Escherichia coli* and *Klebsiella pneumoniae*.

Microbiology departments track the changing sensitivity patterns of their most frequently isolated organisms in a periodic (e.g., quarterly, annually) antibiogram report. The antibiogram report summarizes the sensitivity results of organisms isolated for the first time per year per patient.

Table 5-3 provides an example of an annual antibiogram report. Please note that the antibiogram report results vary according to the organisms and antimicrobials routinely prescribed at a specific hospital. Table 5-3 is an example only and is not necessarily representative of the "typical sensitivity pattern" of the organisms identified at every hospital in the United States.

The antibiogram report is useful in several ways:

1. Clinicians can use the information to guide them in choosing appropriate empirical antimicrobial therapy.
2. The pharmacy department can use the sensitivity results to determine which antimicrobials are effective and should be readily available for the physicians to prescribe through the hospital formulary of medications.
3. The microbiology department, working with the pharmacy, can determine if the selection of antimicrobials per class that are tested should be altered to better reflect the antimicrobials recommended for use.
4. The antimicrobial stewardship committee can use the information to evaluate the effectiveness of their efforts in reducing the overall incidence of resistant organisms isolated from patients. Comparing the current report with previous reports demonstrates the change in sensitivity patterns for the most frequently isolated organisms. If organisms are decreasing in sensitivity to the antimicrobials most frequently prescribed, a change in prescribing practices may help to relieve the antimicrobial selection pressure and reduce the risk of MDROs.

Table 5-1: Antimicrobial Testing

Laboratory Test	Process	Results	Measurement	Interpretation	Key Points
Disk Diffusion (Kirby-Bauer)	• Use a Mueller-Hinton solid agar plate • Inoculate the organism onto the agar plate (organism is diluted to a specified turbidity and spread over the surface of the solid agar plate in all directions to ensure total coverage of the plate's surface) • Place an antimicrobial-impregnated paper disk onto the inoculated plate • Labor: Manual	Measure the zone of inhibition (a cleared circle of "no growth" around the antimicrobial disk where the organism cannot grow due to the antibiotic)	Measure the diameter of area where there is no growth of the organism (zone size) in millimeters (mm) For some bacteriostatic antibiotics, it is necessary to measure the zone of 80% inhibition	Interpret zone sizes, using CLSI-defined criteria, as: S – Sensitive I – Intermediate R – Resistant	Routine testing
Antimicrobial Gradient Diffusion (E-test)	• Use a plate of Mueller-Hinton solid agar • Inoculate organism onto the agar plate (organism is diluted to a specified turbidity and spread over the surface of the solid agar plate in all directions to ensure total coverage of the plate's surface) • Place an antibiotic-impregnated strip with a gradient concentration of antimicrobial agent onto the inoculated plate • Labor: Manual	Measure the zone of inhibition	Read and record the lowest concentration of antimicrobial (µg/mL) that inhibits the growth of the organism around the strip on the agar plate	Interpret the minimum inhibitory concentration (MIC) and record as: S – Sensitive I – Intermediate R – Resistant	Routine testing
Minimum Inhibitory Concentrations (MIC)	• Serial dilutions (e.g., 1:2, 1:4, 1:8) of the antimicrobial agent are inoculated with a liquid suspension of the organism • Labor: Semiautomated or manual broth method	Inhibition of visible growth—there is no turbidity seen in the dilution wells	The well with the lowest (minimum) concentration of the antimicrobial (µg/mL) that inhibits growth is reported	MICs are interpreted according to CLSI or FDA guidelines as: S – Sensitive I – Intermediate R – Resistant	Routine testing
Minimum Bactericidal Concentration (MBC)	• Serial dilutions of antimicrobial agent against actively growing (log-phase) inoculum of the organism • Labor: Manual	Endpoint of growth (calculated from the number of colonies isolated upon subculture of serial dilution tubes above the MIC)	Lowest concentration of antimicrobial (µg/mL) capable of reducing >99.9% of organisms in inoculum upon subculture	MBC is interpreted as: Lowest concentration of antimicrobial that is bactericidal	This test is rarely performed due to the complexity of the testing
Serum Bactericidal Titer (SBT)	• Serial patient serum dilutions against actively growing (log phase) inoculum of organism • Labor: Manual	Endpoint of growth (calculated from the number of colonies isolated upon subculture of serial dilution tubes of the patient's serum that prevented visible growth)	Lowest concentration of serum (µg/mL) capable of reducing >99.9% of organisms in inoculum upon subculture	SBT is interpreted as: Lowest concentration of serum (titer) that is bactericidal to the pathogen	This test is rarely performed due to the complexity of the testing

Table 5-2: Antibiotic Class and Activity

β-lactams

Class	Subclass	Generic Name	Antibiotic Activity Against
Penicillins Action: able to inhibit bacterial enzymes; able to trigger autolytic enzymes that destroy the cell wall; may inhibit RNA synthesis in some bacteria	Penicillin	Penicillin	Non-β-lactamase-producing aerobic Gram positives, some fastidious aerobic Gram negatives, some anaerobes
	Aminopenicillin	Amoxicillin Ampicillin	Additional Gram negatives, including some *Enterobacteriaceae*
	Ureidopenicillin Carboxypenicillin	Piperacillin Carbenicillin Ticarcillin	Expanded list of Gram negatives
	Penicillinase-stable penicillins	Dicloxacillin Flucloxacillin Nafcillin Oxacillin	Penicillinase-producing *Staphylococcus* spp.
β-lactam/β-lactamase inhibitor combinations Action: form an irreversible bond with the β-lactamases leading to a loss of enzyme activity		Amoxicillin-clavulanic acid Ampicillin-sulbactam Piperacillin-tazobactam Ticarcillin-clavulanic acid	Most Gram positives and Gram negatives
Cephems (parenteral) Action: bind to penicillin-binding proteins (PBP), interfering with cell wall synthesis; may trigger autolytic enzymes in the cell	Cephalosporin (narrow spectrum)	Cefazolin Cephradine	Good Gram-positive and modest Gram-negative activity (e.g., *S. pneumoniae*, *S. pyogenes*, some *Enterobacteriaceae*, including many strains of *E. coli*, *Klebsiella* spp., and *Proteus mirabilis*)
	Cephalosporin (expanded spectrum)	Cefuroxime (sodium)	Stable against certain β-lactamases in Gram negatives, therefore have increased activity against them (e.g., some *Enterobacter*, *Serratia*, *Haemophilus* spp., *Neisseria* spp.) None of the expanded spectrum agents is active against *Pseudomonas* spp.
	Cephalosporin (broad spectrum)	Cefoperazone Cefotaxime Ceftazidime Ceftizoxime Ceftriaxone	Generally much less active against Gram-positive cocci, but have increased activity against Gram negatives due to stability against β-lactamases, as well as their ability to penetrate the cell wall of Gram-negative bacilli (e.g., *Enterobacteriaceae* such as *E. coli*, *Proteus* spp., *Klebsiella* spp., with varying activity against *Pseudomonas* spp., *Acinetobacter* spp., *N.gonorrhoeae*)
	Cephalosporin (extended spectrum)	Cefepime Cefpirome Ceftaroline Ceftobiprole	Varied Gram-positive activity (e.g., good against *Staphylococcus* and *Streptococci*; but not enterococci or anaerobes)
	Cephamycin	Cefotetan Cefoxitin	Marked activity against anaerobes (e.g., members of the *B. fragilis* group)
Cephems (oral)	Cephalosporin (narrow spectrum)	Cefadroxil Cephalexin	
	Cephalosporin (expanded spectrum)	Cefaclor Cefprozil Cefuroxime (axetil)	
	Cephalosporin (broad spectrum)	Cefdinir Cefditoren (pivoxil) Cefixime Cefpodoxime (proxetil) Ceftibuten Cephradine	
	Carbacephem	Loracarbef	Active against *H. influenzae* and *Moraxella catarrhalis*

Table 5-2: Antibiotic Class and Activity *(continued)*

β-lactams

Class	Subclass	Generic Name	Antibiotic Activity Against
Monobactams Action: binds to penicillin-binding protein of Gram-negative aerobes, disrupting cell wall synthesis		Aztreonam	Activity only against aerobic Gram negatives; effective against most *Enterobacteriaceae*, including *Enterobacter* spp., *Serratia marcescens*
Penems Action: bind to penicillin-binding proteins of Gram-negative and Gram-positive organisms, causing elongation and lysis	Carbapenem	Doripenem Ertapenem Imipenem Meropenem	Broad-spectrum against non-carbapenemase-producing aerobic and anaerobic Gram positives and Gram negatives; including many *Staphylococci* (not **MRSA**), *Streptococci*, most *Enterobacteriaceae*, and various anaerobic Gram-positive cocci, *Clostridium*, *B. fragilis* group, *Fusobacterium*, and *Prevotella*

Non−β-lactams

Class	Subclass	Generic Name	Antibiotic Activity Against
Aminoglycosides Action: inhibit bacterial protein synthesis by binding irreversibly with the 30S and, in some cases, 50S ribosomal subunit; can be used in synergy with cell-wall active agents against Gram positives		Amikacin Gentamicin Kanamycin Netilmicin Streptomycin Tobramycin	Aerobic Gram negatives and can be used in synergy at high dose levels with cell-wall active agents against Gram positives
Ansamycin Action: interferes with nucleic acid synthesis		Rifampin	Aerobic and anaerobic Gram-positive, Gram-negative, and acid-fast organisms when used in combination therapy
Quinolones Action: targets DNA-gyrase, leading to termination of chromosomal replication and interference with cell division and gene expression	Fluoroquinolone	Ciprofloxacin Gatifloxacin Gemifloxacin Levofloxacin Moxifloxacin Ofloxacin	Many Gram positive and Gram negatives
Folate pathway inhibitors Action: inhibit sequential steps in the bacterial folate pathway		Trimethoprim Trimethoprim-sulfamethoxazole	Some Gram positives and negatives
Fosfomycins Action: inhibits a bacterial cytoplasm enzyme		Fosfomycin	Most Gram positives and Gram negatives found in lower urinary tract infections

Table 5-2: Antibiotic Class and Activity *(continued)*

Non–β-lactams

Class	Subclass	Generic Name	Antibiotic Activity Against
Lipopeptides Action: targets the bacterial cell membrane; activity is strongly influenced by the presence of divalent cations such as iron	Polymyxins	Daptomycin Colistin (polymyxin E) Polymyxin B	Gram positives (daptomycin), aerobic Gram negatives (colistin and polymyxin B)
Macrolides Action: inhibits protein synthesis at the ribosomal level		Azithromycin Clarithromycin Erythromycin	Fastidious Gram negatives and Gram positives
Nitrofurans Action: binds to ribosomal proteins; inhibits synthesis of essential bacterial enzymes; only used to treat urinary tract infections		Nitrofurantoin	Gram positives and Gram negatives causing urinary tract infections, including *S. saprophyticus* and *E. faecalis, Corynebacterium* spp., 90% of *E. coli*
Nitromidazoles Action: once inside the bacterial cell it generates a highly cytotoxic compound that disrupts the cell's DNA		Metronidazole	Various anaerobic bacteria; including *B. fragilis* group, *Fusobacterium* and *Clostridium*, including *C. difficile*; also against protozoa such as *Trichomonas vaginalis, Giardia lamblia,* and *Entamoeba histolytica*
Glycopeptides Action: inhibit cell wall synthesis	Glycopeptide Lipoglycopeptide	Vancomycin Teicoplanin Telavancin	Aerobic Gram positives
Lincosamides Action: bind with the 50S ribosomal subunits and inhibit protein synthesis		Clindamycin	Aerobic Gram-positive cocci and anaerobes
Oxazolidinones Action: inhibit bacterial protein synthesis		Linezolid	Gram positives and mycobacteria
Phenicols Action: inhibit protein synthesis by binding to the 50S ribosomal subunit		Chloramphenicol	Gram positives and Gram negatives
Streptogramins Action: inhibit bacterial protein synthesis		Quinupristin-dalfopristin	Gram positives

Table 5-2: Antibiotic Class and Activity *(continued)*

Non–β-lactams

Class	Subclass	Generic Name	Antibiotic Activity Against
Tetracyclines Action: inhibit protein synthesis		Doxycycline Minocycline Tetracycline	Gram positives and Gram negatives by inhibiting protein synthesis at the ribosomal level
Glycylcyclines Action: inhibit protein synthesis		Tigecycline	Gram positives and Gram negatives that are resistant to tetracyclines

Table 5-3: Example of an Antibiogram

	Number of Isolates Tested	Penicillin	Ceftriaxone (Susceptible)	Oxacillin	Erythromycin	Clindamycin	Vancomycin	TMP/SMZ	Ampicillin	Ampicillin/Sulbactam	Cefazolin	Cefepime	Ceftriaxone	Gentamicin	Gentamicin (High dose)	Tobramycin	Levofloxacin	Ciprofloxacin	Aztreonam	Imipenem	Piperacillin/Tazobactam	Amikacin	Nitrofurantoin (Urine)	Amoxicillin/Clav. Acid (Urine)
Annual Antimicrobic Susceptibility Report for 201X. (Data analysis based on first isolate per patient per year.)																								
Gram positive *S. aureus*—oxacillin resistant	1149/1926 (59%)			0	5	66	100	98															99	
S. aureus—oxacillin sensitive	777/1926 (41%)			100	60	85	100	99															99	
Coagulase negative staph (CNS)	192			31	22	47	100	64															99	
Enterococcus faecium	29						28		14						100								54	
Enterococcus faecalis	95						79		93						47								100	
Gram negative *Enterobacter* spp.—nonurine	150							91		35		95	81	95		87		82	77		81			
Enterobacter spp.—urine	197							82				96	83	95				79					71	
Klebsiella spp.—nonurine	193							88		63	72	95	84	98		96		90	83		85	100		
Klebsiella spp.—urine	682							89			78	96	94	98				91					85	89
Escherichia coli—nonurine	301							83	54	58	87	99	95	93		94		81	96		98	100		
Escherichia coli—urine	3359							83	60		94	100	99	95				88					98	87

References

American Society for Clinical Pathology. Susceptibility testing data—new guidance for developing antibiograms. *Lab Medicine* 2009;40(8):459–462.

Gilbert DN, Moellering, Jr. RC, Eliopoulis GM, et al., eds. *The Sanford Guide to Antimicrobial Therapy 2011*, 41st ed. Sperryville, VA: Antimicrobial Therapy, 2011.

Hindler JF, Barton M, Callihan DR, et al., eds. *Analysis and Presentation of Cumulative Antimicrobial Susceptibility Test Data: Approved Guideline*, 3rd ed. Wayne, PA: Clinical and Laboratory Standards Institute, 2009.

Versalovic J, ed. *Manual of Clinical Microbiology*, 10th ed. Washington, DC: ASM Press, 2011.

Chapter 6

Urinalysis, Fluid Analysis, Chemistry, and Hematology

Nancy Christy, MT, MSHA, CIC

When conducting surveillance and navigating National Healthcare Safety Network (NHSN) surveillance definitions, the infection preventionist (IP) can look to other laboratory disciplines for guidance in interpreting positive cultures. Knowledge of lab tests such as urinalysis, fluid results, chemistry, and hematology can help the IP determine the type of infection and whether it is healthcare-associated. In addition, it is important for IPs to have knowledge of and access to these test results because some lab tests (i.e., liver enzymes) can be requested by state health departments for mandatory reporting.

Urinalysis is very helpful when evaluating for catheter-associated urinary tract infections (UTIs). If the laboratory does not routinely perform Gram stains on urine, the microscopic result can identify whether the urine has bacteria or yeast, especially for urine cultures that grow <100,000 colony-forming units (CFU)/mL. In addition, the urinalysis in conjunction with the urine culture can be instrumental in determining whether a positive blood culture is secondary to a UTI. NHSN states that a positive blood culture with a known pathogen is a bloodstream infection unless it is related to another infection site.

Fluid results, including cerebrospinal fluid (CSF), peritoneal, pleural, and synovial fluid, can aid in determining infections and guide the IP when evaluating bloodstream infections and surgical site infections. The laboratory should send abnormal CSF results—specifically glucose, protein, and cell count—to the infection prevention department to identify possible meningitis.

Chemistry is not often used in infection prevention surveillance. However, the arterial blood gas is very useful in pneumonia identification. The PaO_2 is used for determining worsening gas exchange and is one of the easiest factors of the healthcare-associated pneumonia definition to evaluate. Chemistry may also be helpful for providing additional information to state health departments, depending on the requirements.

The absolute neutrophil count (ANC) can indicate whether a patient is immunocompromised. However, the white blood cell (WBC) count and differential will be the most helpful in determining an infection when using the NHSN pneumonia definition. The CD4 count will help identify immunocompromised patients for PNU3. The WBC count and differential can also identify an infectious process in questionable cases such as bloodstream infections. The differential can sometimes provide clues as to whether there is an infectious process and identify what type (e.g., bacterial versus viral).

The following table provides a general overview of the results and interpretation of tests in urinalysis, fluid, chemistry, and hematology studies. It is by no means a comprehensive list, but is intended to highlight the most common tests and those most utilized for determining infections. It is broken down by the following:

- General category
- Laboratory test
- Indications

- Results
- Specimen
- Frequency (note the majority of this classification is "as needed"; however, there are exceptions)
- Test type
- Interpretation
- Considerations for test or interfering factors
- Key points that relate the test to the appropriate NHSN definition, if applicable

For a more complete list of tests or for those not included on the tables, please refer to the *Lippincott Manual of Nursing Practices Series: Diagnostic Tests*, which is available in most reference libraries, or contact the director of your facility's laboratory for more information.

Table 6-1: Overview of Urinalysis, Fluids, Chemistry, and Hematology Lab Tests

Urinalysis									
Urinalysis (UA)	Appearance	Cloudy or urine with sediment can be an indicator for infection or other abnormal state	Fresh urine is slightly hazy	First morning specimen is best, random specimen can be used (clean catch for accurate results)	As needed	Manually performed by lab	Cloudy: Indicative of a UTI	Cloudy urine can also occur depending on the pH, ingestion of certain types of foods, and fecal contamination	N/A
	Color	The color of the urine can be an indicator of patient's hydration state or an indication of infection	Pale yellow to amber	First morning specimen is best, random specimen can be used (clean catch for accurate results)	As needed	Manually performed by lab	• Colorless urine: large fluid intake, diuretic therapy • Orange: concentrated urine, bilirubin, certain medications • Green: Pseudomonal infection • Pink to red: red blood cells (RBCs), hemoglobin	Drugs and food can cause change in color	N/A
	Odor	• Urine odor can be indicative of a disease • Not usually part of the UA but should be noted	Characteristic aromatic odor	First morning specimen is best, random specimen can be used (clean catch for accurate results)	As needed	Manually performed by lab	Fruity smell: diabetes mellitus Foul: possible UTI	N/A	N/A
	Specific gravity (SG)	• To test the kidney's ability to concentrate urine • Loss of these functions is an indication of renal dysfunction	• Normal hydration and volume = 1.005–1.030 • Concentrated urine: ≤1.025 • Dilute urine: 1.001–1.010 • Infant <2 year: 1.001–1.006	First morning specimen is best, random specimen can be used (clean catch for accurate results)	As needed	Dipstick/reagent strip	• Low SG: Can be indicative of diabetes insipidus, glomerulonephritis, severe renal damage • High SG: Can be diabetes mellitus, nephrosis, dehydration, congestive heart failure (CHF), etc.	Interfering factors can be drugs, temperature, elevated protein, detergent residue, and antibiotics	N/A
	pH	To determine if urine is acidic or alkaline, which is an indicator of how well the kidney is maintaining the body's pH	• pH can vary from 4.6 to 8.0 • The average is 6.0 (acidic)	First morning specimen is best, random specimen can be used (clean catch for accurate results)	As needed	Dipstick/reagent strip	• Several factors increase or decrease pH • Bacteria from a UTI or bacterial contamination can cause the urine to be alkaline	Interfering factors can be food, diet, and drug treatment	N/A

Table 6-1: Overview of Urinalysis, Fluids, Chemistry, and Hematology Lab Tests *(continued)*

Urinalysis									
General Category	Laboratory Test	Indications	Results	Specimen	Frequency	Test Type	Interpretation	Considerations for Test	Key Points
UA *(continued)*	Bilirubin	The presence of bilirubin can aid in the diagnosis and monitoring of treatment for hepatitis and liver damage	Negative	Random or first morning sample is the most common; however, for urobilinogen determination use timed 2-hour volume	As needed	Dipstick/ reagent strip	• Any presence of bilirubin requires further investigation • Besides liver disease, it can be seen with sepsis, obstructive biliary tract disease, and hyperthyroidism	Exposure to light and some drugs can cause erroneous results	N/A
	Blood	Blood in urine is an indicator of damage to the kidney or the urinary tract	Negative	First morning specimen is best, random specimen can be used (clean catch for accurate results)	As needed	Dipstick/ reagent strip	• Presence of free hemoglobin in the urine (hemoglobinuria) indicates rapid destruction of erythrocytes; examples of causes are extensive burns, malaria, hemolytic disorders, disseminated intravascular coagulation (**DIC**), or strenuous exercise • Presence of **RBC**s in the urine (hematuria) is related to trauma or damage to the renal or genitourinary systems; examples of causes are acute UTI, lupus, renal tumors, pyelonephritis, and leukemia to name a few • **M**yoglobin is an excretion of muscle protein from a possible traumatic muscle injury or disorder or poisoning; present when no **RBC**s can be found in the urine and/or other chemical tests	Drugs, menstruation, high doses of vitamin C (ascorbic acid), and prostatic infections are some causes of false-positive results	N/A

Table 6-1: Overview of Urinalysis, Fluids, Chemistry, and Hematology Lab Tests *(continued)*

Urinalysis									
General Category	Laboratory Test	Indications	Results	Specimen	Frequency	Test Type	Interpretation	Considerations for Test	Key Points
UA *(continued)*	Glucose	To test whether the blood glucose levels have exceeded the re-absorption capacity of the tubules (renal threshold)	Negative	• First morning, random (clean catch) is good for screening • For diabetic monitoring, second (double voided) specimen: first morning specimen is discarded; the second is collected and tested; third, postprandial (collected 2 hours after meal)	As needed	Dipstick/ reagent strip or reduction tests	Increase glucose occurs in diabetes mellitus, endocrine disorders, liver and pancreatic diseases	• Large amounts of protein, presence of other nonsugars, and some antibiotics; large amount of ketones can cause a false-negative result • Other false negatives/positives could be stress, excitement, and letting urine sit too long at room temperature	N/A
	Ketone	To test for diabetes (indicator for early diagnosis of ketoacidosis and diabetic coma) or altered carbohydrate metabolism	Negative	First morning specimen is best, random specimen can be used (clean catch for accurate results)	As needed	Dipstick/ reagent strip	Ketonuria in non-diabetic patients can occur during acute illness, severe stress, or strenuous exercises	• Metabolic and dietary conditions can affect the excretion of ketones in the urine • Some drugs and leaving urine standing too long can cause erroneous results	N/A
	Leukocyte esterase	To test for the presence of WBCs in the urine, which can be indicative of an infection	Negative	First morning specimen is best, random specimen can be used (clean catch for accurate results)	As needed	Dipstick/ reagent strip	• Positive results can indicate infection, systemic lupus erythematosus (**SLE**), and tuberculosis infection • This test should be confirmed with a microscopic	• Vaginal discharge, parasites, drug therapies, and strenuous exercise can cause false positives • Large amounts of glucose, protein, and certain drugs can cause false negatives	• Per the NHSN definition, the UA has to be positive if the urine culture is $\geq 10^3$ or $<10^5$ CFU/ mL • For the UA to be positive per NHSN, either the leukocyte esterase, nitrite or the microscopic results (i.e., **WBC**, blood, bacteria) must be present and/or positive

Table 6-1: Overview of Urinalysis, Fluids, Chemistry, and Hematology Lab Tests *(continued)*

Urinalysis									
General Category	Laboratory Test	Indications	Results	Specimen	Frequency	Test Type	Interpretation	Considerations for Test	Key Points
UA *(continued)*	Nitrite	Rapid, indirect test for detecting bacteria in urine	Negative	First morning specimen is best, random specimen can be used (clean catch for accurate results)	As needed	Dipstick/ reagent strip	• A positive result is a clue for performing a urine culture • A negative test should not be used to rule out bacteriuria because some organisms such as staphylococci and streptococci do not convert nitrate to nitrite or if a first morning specimen is not used	Bilirubin, ascorbic acid, and leaving the urine at room temperature too long will cause erroneous results	• Per the NHSN definition, the UA has to be positive if the urine culture is $\geq 10^3$ or $<10^5$ CFU/ mL • For the UA to be positive per NHSN, either the leukocyte esterase, nitrite, or the microscopic results (i.e., WBC, blood, bacteria) must be present and/or positive
	Protein	Presence of protein is an important indication of renal disease	Negative	First morning specimen is best, random specimen can be used (clean catch for accurate results)	As needed	Dipstick/ reagent strip	• Proteinuria can occur because of glomerular damage or diminished tubular reabsorption • The results can vary so any protein in urine is considered to be abnormal • The level does not indicate the severity of disease	• Exercise and fever can also lead to increased protein in the urine • If more than trace protein is found in the urine, a 24-hour protein can be done	• Proteinuria can occur in acute infection and septicemia • Large numbers of WBC with proteinuria usually indicate an infection somewhere in the urinary tract
	Urine crystals	The presence of crystals can be associated with partial or complete obstruction of urine flow	Normal crystals seen: amorphous, sodium urate, calcium oxalate, hippuric acid, calcium carbonate, ammonium biurate, calcium phosphate, amorphous phosphates	First morning specimen is best, random specimen can be used (clean catch for accurate results)	As requested or to verify positive dipstick	Microscopic	Abnormal crystals: uric acid, cystine, cholesterol, leucine, bilirubin, calcium oxalate (in large quantities only), and triple phosphate	• Exposing urine to low or room temperature can cause formation or reabsorption of crystals • Radiographic dye may cause crystals in dehydrated patients	N/A

Table 6-1: Overview of Urinalysis, Fluids, Chemistry, and Hematology Lab Tests *(continued)*

Urinalysis									
General Category	Laboratory Test	Indications	Results	Specimen	Frequency	Test Type	Interpretation	Considerations for Test	Key Points
UA *(continued)*	Urine RBCs and RBCs casts	Indicator of serious renal disease	• RBCs: 0–3/ high-power field (hpf) • RBC casts: 0/ low-power field (lpf)	First morning specimen is best, random specimen can be used (clean catch for accurate results)	As requested or to verify positive dipstick	Microscopic	• RBCs in the urine can be from several things; for IP review, it could mean malaria, renal tuberculosis, and acute febrile episodes • RBC casts can either be from a hemorrhage in the nephron or acute inflammatory or vascular disorders • They can also be seen in acute bacterial endocarditis	Strenuous exercise, heavy smoking, some drugs, alkaline urine, and traumatic catheterization can interfere with the test	• When looking at WBCs for infection, review presence or amount of RBCs • Of note, large amounts of WBCs and RBCs could indicate a noninfectious inflammatory disease rather than an infection
	Urine WBCs and WBC casts	Indicates inflammation in the genitourinary system or an infection	• WBCs: 0–4/ hpf • Normal women may have slightly higher WBCs due to contamination with vaginal contents during collection • WBC casts: 0/lpf	First morning specimen is best, random specimen can be used (clean catch for accurate results)	As requested or to verify positive dipstick	Microscopic	• WBCs in the urine can indicate a UTI, appendicitis, bladder tumors, tuberculosis, and SLE • WBC casts show up in renal parenchymal infections (most common is pyelonephritis)	Vaginal discharge can interfere with test	• Per the NHSN definition, the UA has to be positive if the urine culture is $\geq 10^3$ or $<10^5$ CFU/ mL • For the UA to be positive per NHSN, either the leukocyte esterase, nitrite, or the microscopic results (i.e., WBC, blood, bacteria) must be present and/or positive

Table 6-1: Overview of Urinalysis, Fluids, Chemistry, and Hematology Lab Tests *(continued)*

Urinalysis									
General Category	Laboratory Test	Indications	Results	Specimen	Frequency	Test Type	Interpretation	Considerations for Test	Key Points
UA *(continued)*	Urine epithelial cells and epithelial casts	To indicate the health of the renal tubules, and could indicate poisoning	• Renal tubule epithelial cells: 0–3/hpf • Squamous epithelial cells: normal • Renal tubule epithelial casts: 0	First morning specimen is best, random specimen can be used (clean catch for accurate results)	As requested or to verify positive dipstick	Microscopic	• Epithelial cell casts indicate exposure to toxic agents or viruses • Renal tubular epithelial cells can be seen in viral infections (i.e., cytomegalovirus [CMV]), poisoning from heavy metals, and impending allograft rejection	N/A	N/A
	Urine hyaline casts	To ascertain any possible damage to the glomerular capillary membrane	Occasional, 0–2/lpf	First morning specimen is best, random specimen can be used (clean catch for accurate results)	As requested or to verify positive dipstick	Microscopic	Hyaline casts are not clinically associated with any clinical disorder	N/A	N/A
	Urine granular casts	Presence can indicate health of renal tubules	Occasional, 0–2/lpf	First morning specimen is best, random specimen can be used (clean catch for accurate results)	As requested or to verify positive dipstick	Microscopic	• Granular casts can be found in acute tubular necrosis, advanced glomerulonephritis, pyelonephritis, and malignant nephrosclerosis • Presence with hyaline casts can indicate strenuous exercise or stress	N/A	N/A
	Urine waxy cast or broad casts (renal failure casts) and fatty casts	Can indicate renal failure	Negative	First morning specimen is best, random specimen can be used (clean catch for accurate results)	As requested or to verify positive dipstick	Microscopic	• Broad and waxy casts occur in several diseases, most notably severe renal failure and renal allograft rejection • Fatty casts are found in chronic disorders such as lupus and chronic glomerulonephritis • Can also be seen in toxic renal poisoning	N/A	N/A

Table 6-1: Overview of Urinalysis, Fluids, Chemistry, and Hematology Lab Tests *(continued)*

Urinalysis									
General Category	Laboratory Test	Indications	Results	Specimen	Frequency	Test Type	Interpretation	Considerations for Test	Key Points
UA *(continued)*	Osmolality	An exact measurement of renal concentration; it is a more accurate measurement of renal function than SG	Urine to serum ratio is 1:1 to 3:1. 50–1,200 mOsm/kg of H_2O	Random sample	As needed	Analyzed by lab	• When osmolality is increased, it can be indicative of several diseases such as Addison disease, dehydration, CHF, and hyponatremia • When osmolality is decreased, it can be indicative of acute renal failure, diabetes insipidus, and compulsive water drinking	N/A	N/A
24-hour timed urine specimen	Urine chloride	Indicates the state of the electrolyte balance	• Adults: 140–250 mEq/24 hours • Children <6: 15–40 mEq/24 hours • Children 10–14: 64–176 mEq/24 hours	Refrigerate during collection	As needed	Analyzed by lab	• Decreased urine chloride can come from vomiting, diarrhea, excessive sweating, gastric suction, Addison disease, metabolic alkalosis, etc. • Increased chloride can occur with increased salt intake, adrenocortical insufficiency, potassium depletion, Barter syndrome, and salt-losing nephritis	Antibiotic therapy, dietary intake, ingestion of licorice, ammonium chloride administration, and excessive infusion of normal saline can interfere with test	N/A
	Urine sodium	To measure one aspect of the electrolyte balance that is managed by the kidneys (useful for diagnosis of renal, adrenal, water, and acid-base imbalances)	• Adults: 40–220 mEq/24 hour • Children: 41–115 mEq/24 hours	Refrigerate during collection	As needed	Analyzed by lab	• Increased urine sodium can be seen in various disorders such as Addison disease, diabetic acidosis, Barter syndrome • Decreased urine sodium most notably seen in CHF, Cushing disease, and primary aldosteronism	Caffeine intake, diuretic therapy, dehydration, use of corticosteroids, propranolol, and premenstrual water retention can affect results	N/A

Table 6-1: Overview of Urinalysis, Fluids, Chemistry, and Hematology Lab Tests *(continued)*

Urinalysis									
General Category	Laboratory Test	Indications	Results	Specimen	Frequency	Test Type	Interpretation	Considerations for Test	Key Points
24-hour timed urine specimen *(continued)*	Urine potassium	• To test for renal and adrenal disorders • Also useful with water and acid-base imbalances	• Adult: 25–125 mEq/24 hours • Child: 10–60 mEq/24 hours	Refrigerate during collection	As needed	Analyzed by lab	• Increased urine potassium can be seen in various disorders, most notably seen in primary renal disease, starvation, Cushing syndrome, and onset of metabolic alkalosis • Decreased urine potassium can be seen in Addison disease and severe renal disease	Values are diet-dependent cortisone, antibiotics, licorice, and glucose intravenous (IV) infusion are some interfering factors	N/A
	Uric acid	To evaluate uric acid metabolism and evaluate stone formation and nephrolithiasis	• Normal diet: 250–750 mg/24 hours • With purine-free diet: <400 mg/24 hours With high purine diet: <1000 mg/24 hours	Refrigerate during collection	As needed	Analyzed by lab	• Increased uric acid occurs most notably in gout, chronic myelogenous leukemia, polycythemia vera, viral hepatitis, and sickle cell anemia • Decreased uric acid can be found in chronic kidney disease, xanthinuria, folic acid deficiency, and lead toxicity	Interfering factors can be diuretics, vitamin C, warfarin, X-ray contrast media, and strenuous exercise	N/A

Fluids									
Cerebrospinal fluid (CSF)	Pressure	To detect cranial pressure	50–180 mm H_2O	N/A	As needed	Initial pressure taken by doctor at initial insertion and final removal of needle	• Increase: increased intracranial pressure due to meningitis, cerebral edema, and intracranial tumors, abscess, or lesions • Decrease: severe dehydration and obstruction in spinal subarachnoid above puncture site	Slight elevation of CSF pressure may occur in an anxious patient (specifically breath holding or tensing muscles)	N/A

Table 6-1: Overview of Urinalysis, Fluids, Chemistry, and Hematology Lab Tests *(continued)*

Fluids									
General Category	Laboratory Test	Indications	Results	Specimen	Frequency	Test Type	Interpretation	Considerations for Test	Key Points
CSF *(continued)*	Appearance	To aid in detection of infection, hemorrhage, and obstruction	Clear and colorless	CSF	As needed	Manual observation	• Cloudy: infection • Xanthochromic (yellow discoloration) or bloody: hemorrhage, spinal cord obstruction, or traumatic tap • Brown, orange, or yellow: elevated protein, RBC breakdown	• A traumatic lumbar puncture can change the appearance • If sample is bloody in tubes 1 and 2 more than 3 or 4 then the bloody sample appearance is probably due to a traumatic lumbar puncture	N/A
	Protein	To aid in detection of meningitis, brain abscess, multiple sclerosis (MS), tumors, and other processes causing neoplastic disease	15–50 mg/dL	CSF	As needed	Automated	• Increase: bacterial meningitis, tumors, trauma, diabetes mellitus, polyneuritis, and blood in CSF • Decrease: rapid CSF production	A traumatic tap will invalidate the protein results (see appearance)	• Part of the NHSN MEN (meningitis or ventriculitis) definition: increase in protein and increased WBC and/ or decreased glucose
	Albumin and immunoglobulin G (IgG)	In conjunction with serum levels of albumin and IgG, this test helps dictate damage to the blood–central nervous system (CNS) barrier	• Albumin: 10–35 mg/dL or 1.5–5.3 μmol/L • IgG: <4.0 mg/dL or <40 mg/L • CSF IgG index: <0.60	CSF	As needed	Automated	• The CSF serum albumin index <9.0: intact blood–brain barrier 9-14: slight impairment to the barrier 14-30: moderate impairment of the barrier >30: severe impairment • Increased albumin: Guillain-Barré syndrome and other infectious diseases (e.g., tularemia and bacterial meningitis) • Increased CSF IgG index: MS and neurosyphilis	A traumatic tap will invalidate the results (see appearance)	N/A

Table 6-1: Overview of Urinalysis, Fluids, Chemistry, and Hematology Lab Tests *(continued)*

Fluids									
General Category	Laboratory Test	Indications	Results	Specimen	Frequency	Test Type	Interpretation	Considerations for Test	Key Points
CSF *(continued)*	Glucose	To aid in the detection of infection, systemic hyperglycemia, or hemorrhage	50–80 mg/dL	CSF	As needed	Automated	• Increase: systemic hyperglycemia • Decrease: systemic hypoglycemia, bacterial or fungal infection, meningitis, mumps, post- subarachnoid hemorrhage	A traumatic tap may produce misleading results due to the presence of glucose in blood	• Part of the NHSN MEN (meningitis or ventriculitis) definition: increase in protein and increased WBC and/ or decreased glucose • Note: viral meningitis will usually have a normal glucose, whereas bacterial meningitis will have a decreased glucose
	Cell count	To aid in the detection of infection, neurologic diseases, or hemorrhage	• WBCs: 0–5/ hpf • RBCs: 0/hpf	CSF	As needed	Automated or performed by MT manually	• Increase in WBC: neutrophils can be seen in bacterial or early viral meningitis; monocytes in chronic bacterial or viral meningitis; lymphocytes in viral meningitis; blast forms in acute leukemia • Increase in RBC: hemorrhage or traumatic lumbar puncture	A traumatic tap may produce misleading results due to presence of blood in CSF (see appearance)	Part of the NHSN MEN (meningitis or ventriculitis) definition: increase in protein and increased WBC and/ or decreased glucose
	Chloride	To detect infection in meninges	11–130 mEq/L	CSF	As needed	Automated	Decrease: infected meninges		N/A
	Venereal Disease Research Laboratory (VDRL)	To identify neurosyphilis	Negative	CSF	As needed		Positive: neurosyphilis		N/A

Table 6-1: Overview of Urinalysis, Fluids, Chemistry, and Hematology Lab Tests *(continued)*

Fluids									
General Category	Laboratory Test	Indications	Results	Specimen	Frequency	Test Type	Interpretation	Considerations for Test	Key Points
Arthrocentesis	Color	To assess joints for an infection or inflammatory response	Clear	Synovial fluid	As needed	Manual observation	Septic: variable, may be purulent		N/A
	Clarity/ appearance	To assess joints for an infection or inflammatory response	Transparent	Synovial fluid	As needed	Manual observation	Septic: opaque		N/A
	Cell count	To assess joints for an infection or inflammatory response	• WBCs: 200 mm^3 • Neutrophils (%): <25	Synovial fluid	As needed	Manual count performed by lab	• Septic: >50,000 mm^3 and >75% of neutrophils usually • Refer to laboratory for normal ranges	Specimen contamination and/or acid diluents may affect results	Part of the following NHSN definitions: JNT: WBC plus glucose compatible with infection and no underlying rheumatologic disorder; also used to classify organ-space surgical site infection (SSI)
	Glucose	To assess joints for an infection, or inflammatory response	Usually 20% less than serum glucose	Synovial fluid; in addition, a fasting serum glucose (at least 6–8 hours) should be performed for comparison	As needed	Automated	Septic arthritis: synovial fluid glucose level 40 mg/dL less than the serum level (ratio <0.5)	Specimen contamination or patient did not follow diet restrictions (fasting)	Part of the following NHSN definitions: JNT: WBC plus glucose compatible with infection and no underlying rheumatologic disorder; also used to classify organ-space SSI

Table 6-1: Overview of Urinalysis, Fluids, Chemistry, and Hematology Lab Tests *(continued)*

Fluids									
General Category	Laboratory Test	Indications	Results	Specimen	Frequency	Test Type	Interpretation	Considerations for Test	Key Points
Peritoneal analysis	Gross appearance	To identify abdominal trauma or determine the cause of ascites	Sterile, odorless color is clear to pale yellow; amounts are usually <50 mL	Fluid collected from area below umbilicus	As needed	Manual observation	• Cloudy: bacterial infection, ruptured bowel, pancreatitis, infarcted intestine, or appendicitis • Bloody: benign or malignant tumor, hemorrhagic pancreatitis or traumatic tap • Bile-stained, green: ruptured gallbladder, acute pancreatitis, or a perforated intestine or duodenal ulcer • Milk colored: thoracic duct that is damaged or blocked by a tumor, lymphoma, tuberculosis, parasitic infestation, adhesion, or hepatic cirrhosis	Contamination of the specimen with blood, bile, urine, or stool	N/A
	RBCs	To identify abdominal trauma or determine the cause of ascites	None	Fluid collected from area below umbilicus	As needed	Manual cell count	• RBC >100/µL indicates neoplasm or tuberculosis • RBC >100,000/µL indicates intra-abdominal trauma	Contamination of the specimen with blood	N/A

Table 6-1: Overview of Urinalysis, Fluids, Chemistry, and Hematology Lab Tests *(continued)*

Fluids									
General Category	Laboratory Test	Indications	Results	Specimen	Frequency	Test Type	Interpretation	Considerations for Test	Key Points
Peritoneal analysis *(continued)*	WBCs	To identify abdominal trauma or determine the cause of ascites	<300/µL	Fluid collected from area below umbilicus	As needed	Manual cell count	• WBC: elevated (≥300/µL) with more than 25% neutrophils occurs in 90% of patients with spontaneous bacterial peritonitis and 50% of those with cirrhosis • A high percentage of the following WBCs represents the following diseases: Neutrophils: bacterial peritonitis or cirrhosis Lymphocytes: tuberculosis or chylous ascites Mesothelial cells: tuberculosis	Contamination of the specimen with blood	N/A
	Protein	To identify abdominal trauma or determine the cause of ascites	0.3 to 4.1 g/dL	Fluid collected from area below umbilicus	As needed	Automated	• Protein levels > 3 g/dL: malignancy • Protein levels >4 g/dL: tuberculosis	Contamination of the specimen with blood	N/A
	Amylase	To identify abdominal trauma or determine the cause of ascites	138 to 404 U/L	Fluid collected from area below umbilicus	As needed	Automated	Elevated amylase: pancreatic trauma, pancreatic pseudocyst, or acute pancreatitis or intestinal necrosis	Contamination of the specimen with blood	N/A
	Ammonia	To identify abdominal trauma or determine the cause of ascites	<50 µg/dL	Fluid collected from area below umbilicus	As needed	Automated	Ammonia levels that are twice the normal serum levels of amylase: ruptured or strangulated large and small intestine, ruptured ulcer or an appendix	Contamination of the specimen with blood	N/A

Table 6-1: Overview of Urinalysis, Fluids, Chemistry, and Hematology Lab Tests *(continued)*

Fluids									
General Category	Laboratory Test	Indications	Results	Specimen	Frequency	Test Type	Interpretation	Considerations for Test	Key Points
Peritoneal analysis *(continued)*	Alkaline phosphatase	To identify abdominal trauma or determine the cause of ascites	• Men > age 18: 90–239 U/L • Women < age 45: 76–196 U/L • Women > age 45: 87–250 U/L	Fluid collected from area below umbilicus	As needed	Automated	Alkaline phosphatase more than twice normal serum levels: ruptured or strangulated small intestines	Contamination of the specimen with blood	N/A
Thoracentesis	Gross appearance	Evaluate pleural effusion for infection	Clear, straw colored, and odorless	Pleural fluid from thoracic wall	As needed	Manual observation	• Blood: may indicate traumatic tap or hemothorax • Cloudy or pus filled: infection or necrotic tissue • Serosanguinous: malignant tumor • Putrid odor: anaerobic empyema	N/A	N/A
	Glucose	Evaluate pleural effusion for infection	Similar to serum glucose ranges	Pleural fluid from thoracic wall	As needed	Automated	Low levels or <60 mg/dL or a pleural fluid glucose and serum glucose ratio <0.5: rheumatoid pleurisy, tuberculosis pleurisy, lupus pleurisy, parapneumonic empyema, or effusion	N/A	N/A

Table 6-1: Overview of Urinalysis, Fluids, Chemistry, and Hematology Lab Tests *(continued)*

Fluids									
General Category	Laboratory Test	Indications	Results	Specimen	Frequency	Test Type	Interpretation	Considerations for Test	Key Points
Thoracentesis *(continued)*	Protein	Used in determining whether pleural fluid is exudate or transudate	Not available (no established reference values)	Pleural fluid from thoracic wall	As needed	Automated	• Pleural fluid protein and serum protein ratio of >0.5 or a pleural fluid protein of >2.9 g/dL • Factors that determine if it is an exudate need at least one of protein, lactate dehydrogenase (LDH), or cholesterol; if none of these factors are "positive" then it is transudate • Exudate diseases include (not complete): bacterial pneumonia, parasites, atypical pneumonia, hepatic abscess, pancreatitis, and pulmonary embolism • If transudate does not meet the criteria, see LDH, and cholesterol; may be malignancy, pulmonary embolism, sarcoidosis, congenital heart failure, and atelectasis	N/A	N/A
	Lactate dehydrogenase (LDH)	Used in determining whether pleural fluid is exudate or transudate	Not available (no established reference values)	Pleural fluid from thoracic wall	As needed	Automated	• Pleural fluid LDH and serum LDH ratio of >0.6 or pleural fluid LDH result >0.45 of upper levels of normal serum LDH • Factors that determine if it is an exudate: need at least one of protein, LDH, or cholesterol; if none of these factors are "positive" then it is transudate • See Protein (above) for common diseases	N/A	N/A

Table 6-1: Overview of Urinalysis, Fluids, Chemistry, and Hematology Lab Tests *(continued)*

Fluids									
General Category	Laboratory Test	Indications	Results	Specimen	Frequency	Test Type	Interpretation	Considerations for Test	Key Points
Thoracentesis *(continued)*	Cholesterol	Used in determining whether pleural fluid is exudate or transudate	Not available (no established reference values)	Pleural fluid from thoracic wall	As needed	Automated	• Pleural fluid cholesterol and serum cholesterol ratio of >0.3 or pleural fluid cholesterol result of 45 mg/dL • Factors that determine if it is an exudate: need at least one of protein, LDH, or cholesterol; if none of these factors are "positive" then it is transudate • See Protein (above) for common diseases	N/A	N/A
	Amylase	Aid in diagnosing the source of excess pleural fluid	Not available (no established reference values)	Pleural fluid from thoracic wall	As needed	Automated	Elevated pleural effusion alpha-amylase suggests acute pancreatitis as the cause of the effusion	N/A	N/A
	WBC	Evaluate pleural effusion for infection	<1,000/mm^3	Pleural fluid from thoracic wall	As needed	Manual cell count	Elevated levels of neutrophils: septic, inflammation lymphocytes- tuberculosis, fungal or viral effusions	N/A	N/A

Chemistry									
Electrolyte panel	Na (sodium)	Evaluate the fluid-electrolyte and acid-base balance and related neuromuscular, renal, and adrenal functions	135–145 mEq/L	3–4 mL clot-activator tube	As needed	Automated	• Low levels of sodium: dehydration from excessive sweating, gastrointestinal (GI) suctioning, diuretic therapy, and burns • Higher levels of sodium: inadequate water intake, sodium retention (i.e., aldosteronism), and excessive sodium intake	Diuretics, drugs such as chlorpropamide or corticosteroids, and antihypertensive can affect sodium	N/A

Table 6-1: Overview of Urinalysis, Fluids, Chemistry, and Hematology Lab Tests *(continued)*

Chemistry									
General Category	Laboratory Test	Indications	Results	Specimen	Frequency	Test Type	Interpretation	Considerations for Test	Key Points
Electrolyte panel *(continued)*	K (potassium)	Used in evaluating excess or depletion of potassium which can aid in monitoring renal function, acid-base balance, and glucose metabolism	3.5–5 mEq/L	3–4 mL clot-activator tube	As needed	Automated	• High serum potassium (hyperkalemia): burn or crush injuries, diabetic ketoacidosis, transfusions, and myocardial infarction • Low potassium levels (hypokalemia): Cushing syndrome, long-term diuretic therapy, vomiting, diarrhea, and excessive licorice ingestion	Renal toxicity from certain drugs, excessive or rapid potassium infusion, and some IV therapy (insulin or glucose as well)	N/A
	Cl (chlorine)	Aids in detecting the acid-base imbalance and used to evaluate fluid status and extracellular cation-anion balance	100–108 mEq/L	3–4 mL clot-activator tube	As needed	Automated	• Increased levels: may be from several factors such as severe dehydration, renal shutdown, head injury, and primary aldosteronism • Decreased levels: low sodium and potassium levels due to vomiting, gastric suctioning, intestinal fistula, chronic renal failure, Addison disease, heart failure, or edema	N/A	N/A
	CO$_2$ (carbon dioxide)	Assesses bicarbonate levels and used to evaluate the acid-base balance and pH	22–26 mEq/L	3–4 mL clot-activator tube	As needed	Automated	• High CO$_2$ levels: may occur in metabolic alkalosis, respiratory acidosis, primary aldosteronism, and Cushing syndrome • Low CO$_2$ levels: seen in metabolic acidosis	Excessive use of diuretics, alkali and licorice ingestion, ingestion of ethylene or methyl alcohol, or other drugs can affect CO$_2$	N/A

Table 6-1: Overview of Urinalysis, Fluids, Chemistry, and Hematology Lab Tests *(continued)*

Chemistry									
General Category	Laboratory Test	Indications	Results	Specimen	Frequency	Test Type	Interpretation	Considerations for Test	Key Points
Electrolyte panel *(continued)*	Mg (magnesium)	Evaluates electrolyte status, neuromuscular and renal function	1.3–2.1 mg/dL	3–4 mL clot-activator tube	As needed	Automated	• Increased magnesium: results from renal failure and adrenal insufficiency • Decreased magnesium: can be from several factors such as chronic alcoholism, malabsorption syndrome, diarrhea, prolonged bowel or gastric aspiration, acute pancreatitis, and severe burns	Drugs such as antacids, lithium, alcohol, aminoglycosides, and prolonged IV without magnesium can affect magnesium	N/A
Cardiac markers	Cardiac troponin	Used to diagnose acute myocardial infarction (AMI) and evaluate chest pain	• Detectable levels are considered positive • Refer to individual laboratory values	7 mL clot-activator tube	As needed	Automated	Elevated levels are seen within 1 hour of myocardial cell injury	Surgical procedures, cardiotoxic drugs, and sustained vigorous exercise can affect troponin levels	N/A
	Creatine kinase (CK)	Used to diagnose AMI, evaluate chest pain, and detect early dermatomyositis and musculoskeletal disorders	• Total CK in men: 55–170 U/L • Total CK in women: 30–135 U/L	4 mL tube without additives	As needed	Automated	• CK-BB: may indicate brain tissue injury, malignant tumors, severe shock, or renal failure • CK-MB: fluctuates depending on how many hours have passed since AMI or cardiac surgery; there may be a mild increase in CK-MB with serious skeletal muscle injury • CK-MM: increases following skeletal muscle damage from trauma, surgery, dermatomyositis, and muscular dystrophy • Total CK: may increase with severe hypokalemia, carbon monoxide poisoning, malignant hyperthermia, and alcoholic cardiomyopathy	Surgery, various drugs, alcohol, lithium, cardioversion, vigorous exercise, and trauma can interfere with CK	N/A

Table 6-1: Overview of Urinalysis, Fluids, Chemistry, and Hematology Lab Tests *(continued)*

Chemistry									
General Category	Laboratory Test	Indications	Results	Specimen	Frequency	Test Type	Interpretation	Considerations for Test	Key Points
Cardiac markers *(continued)*	Homocysteine	One of the tests to evaluate risk factors for atherosclerotic vascular disease and inborn metabolism errors of B6, B12, methionine, and folate	4–17 µmol/L	Fast for 12 hours prior to test; collect in a 5-mL tube with EDTA	As needed	Automated	• Some biochemical deficiencies are associated with low homocysteine levels • Elevated homocysteine levels are associated with a higher incidence of atherosclerotic vascular disease	Low intake of B vitamins, contraceptives, carbamazepine, renal impairment, and smoking are some interfering factors	N/A
	LDH	Aids in diagnosing AMI, and depending on the isoenzyme can be used with diagnosing hepatic, pulmonary, and erythrocyte damage	Total LDH ranges from 71–207 U/L	3–4 mL clot-activator tube	As needed	Automated	• LDH has many isoenzymes (LD_1 through LD_5), and it varies by disease • For a complete breakdown, see *Lippincott Manual of Nursing Practices Series: Diagnostic Tests*	Pregnancy, prosthetic heart valve, alcohol, anabolic steroids, and opioids can affect results	N/A
Kidney functions	Blood urea nitrogen (BUN)	Used for assessing hydration or diagnosis of renal disease	8–20 mg/dL	3–4 mL clot-activator tube	As needed	Automated	• Low levels: severe liver damage, malnutrition, and excess hydration • High levels: renal disease, urinary tract obstruction, and burns	Diet, pregnancy, IV feedings can increase or decrease BUN levels	N/A
	Phosphorus	Evaluate kidney disease and vitamin D intake	2.5–4.5 mg/100 mL	3–4 mL clot-activator tube	As needed	Automated	• Increased phosphorus: hypoparathyroidism, kidney disease, or excessive intake of vitamin D • Decreased phosphorus: hyperthyroidism, rickets, and some kidney diseases	Hemolysis, drugs, seasonal variations, and laxatives can increase or decrease BUN levels	N/A
	Creatinine	Assess glomerular filtration and screen for renal damage	• Men: 0.8–1.2 mg/dL • Women: 0.6–0.9 mg/dL	3–4 mL clot-activator tube	As needed	Automated	• Elevated creatinine: indicates renal disease that has damaged ≥50% or more of the nephrons • May also be associated with gigantism and acromegaly	High levels of ascorbic acid, barbiturates, diuretics, large muscle mass can influence creatinine levels	N/A

Table 6-1: Overview of Urinalysis, Fluids, Chemistry, and Hematology Lab Tests *(continued)*

Chemistry									
General Category	Laboratory Test	Indications	Results	Specimen	Frequency	Test Type	Interpretation	Considerations for Test	Key Points
Kidney functions *(continued)*	Uric acid	Diagnostic for gout and to detect renal dysfunction	• Men: 3.4–7 mg/dL • Women: 2.3–6 mg/dL	Fast 8 hours before test and draw in 3–4 mL clot-activator tube	As needed	Automated	• Elevated uric acid: gout, impaired kidney function, heart failure, glycogen storage disease, infections, hemolytic and sickle cell anemia, polycythemia, neoplasms, and psoriasis • Low uric acid: defective tubular absorption or acute hepatic atrophy	• Usually performed in conjunction with urine uric acid • Drugs such as aspirin, pyrazinamide, alcohol abuse, and starvation may affect results	N/A
Lipids	Cholesterol	Evaluates the risk for arthrosclerosis, myocardial occlusion, and coronary arterial occlusion	• Vary with age, diet, sex, and region • Adults fasting: Desirable: 140–199 mg/dL Borderline: 200–239 mg/dL High: >240 mg/dL • Children (12–18) Desirable: <170 mg/dL Borderline: 170–199 mg/dL High: >200 mg/dL	5 mL venous blood specimen	As needed	Automated	• Elevated: helps to classify coronary heart disease risk but can also be seen in nephrotic syndrome, chronic renal failure, alcoholism, and poorly controlled diabetes • Decreased cholesterol levels: severe hepatocellular disease, hyperthyroidism, severe burns, inflammation, conditions of acute illness or infection, and chronic obstructive pulmonary disease (COPD)	Estrogens, drugs, seasonal effects, positional variants, and EDTA can affect results	N/A
	Triglycerides	Helps establish risk of coronary artery disease (CAD) and early identification of hyperlipidemia	• Men: 44–180 mg/dL • Women: 11–190 mg/dL	4 mL EDTA tube	As needed	Automated	• Elevated: biliary obstruction, diabetes mellitus, nephrotic syndrome, endocrinopathies, or excessive alcohol • Decreased: rare and occurs mainly in malnutrition and abetalipoproteinemia	• Additional tests will be needed for definitive diagnosis • Various drugs affect results (examples): antilipemics, cholestyramine, alcohol, corticosteroids, estrogen, contraceptives, and niacin	N/A

Table 6-1: Overview of Urinalysis, Fluids, Chemistry, and Hematology Lab Tests *(continued)*

Chemistry									
General Category	Laboratory Test	Indications	Results	Specimen	Frequency	Test Type	Interpretation	Considerations for Test	Key Points
Lipids *(continued)*	Lipoprotein electrophoresis (LDL, HDL, and lipoprotein)	Fractionation tests used to isolate and measure types of cholesterol which helps assess the risk of CAD and the type of hyper- or hypolipoproteinemia	• Laboratory tests may vary by geographic area, age, or ethic group • Check with local laboratory for value ranges	• Fast 12–14 hours before test • 4–7 mL EDTA tube	As needed	Automated	• Elevated LDL: increases risk of CAD • Elevated HDL: chronic hepatitis, early-stage primary biliary cirrhosis, and alcohol consumption • Hyperlipoproteinemias and hyperlipoproteinemias identification are dependent on electrophoretic pattern • Please see *Lippincott Manual of Nursing Practice Series: Diagnostic Tests* for complete list of diseases	Various factors can affect results (not inclusive) such as fever, heparin administration, antilipemics, alcohol, estrogens, presence of bilirubin	N/A
Liver function	Total protein	Aids in diagnosis of hepatic disease, protein deficiency, renal disorders, GI and neoplastic disease	6.4–8.3 g/dL	7 mL clot-activator tube	As needed	Automated	• Elevated protein levels: chronic inflammatory disease, dehydration, chronic infections, vomiting, and diarrhea • Decreased protein levels: heart failure, hepatic dysfunction, hemorrhage, severe burns, and uncontrolled diabetes mellitus	Cytotoxic drugs or pregnancy can affect results	N/A
	Globulin	Aids in diagnosis of hepatic disease, protein deficiency, renal disorders, GI and neoplastic disease	• Depends on fraction • Alpha₁: 0.1–0.3 g/dL • Alpha₂: 0.6–1 g/dL • Beta: 0.7–1.1 g/dL • Gamma: 0.8–1.6 g/dL	8 mL clot-activator tube	As needed	Automated	• Increased globulin levels: chronic syphilis, collagen diseases, rheumatoid arthritis, subacute bacterial endocarditis, and tuberculosis • Decreased globulin levels: GI disease, heart failure, severe burns, surgical and traumatic shock	N/A	N/A

Table 6-1: Overview of Urinalysis, Fluids, Chemistry, and Hematology Lab Tests *(continued)*

Chemistry									
General Category	Laboratory Test	Indications	Results	Specimen	Frequency	Test Type	Interpretation	Considerations for Test	Key Points
Liver function *(continued)*	Albumin	Aids in diagnosis of hepatic disease, protein deficiency, renal disorders, GI and neoplastic disease	3.5–5 g/dL	7 mL clot-activator tube	As needed	Automated	• Increased albumin: seen in multiple myelomas • Decreased levels of albumin: diarrhea, acute cholecystitis, hepatic disease, Hodgkin disease, and peptic ulcer	N/A	N/A
	Total bilirubin	Evaluates liver function, monitors jaundice, and aids in diagnosis of biliary obstruction of hemolytic anemia • Also used for treatment therapy for neonates	• Direct serum: <0.5 mg/dL • Indirect serum: 1.1 mg/dL • Neonates: 2–12 mg/dL	3–4 mL clot-activator tube	As needed	Automated	• Elevated indirect serum bilirubin levels: hepatic damage, severe hemolytic anemia, and congenital enzyme deficiencies • Elevated direct serum bilirubin levels: biliary obstruction and chronic hepatic damage • In neonates, total bilirubin levels ≥15 mg/dL: indicates the need for an exchange transfusion	Contraceptives, aminoglycosides, barbiturates, and moderate alcohol intake can affect the results	N/A
	Alkaline phosphatase (ALP)	Useful in testing for metabolic bone disease	30–85 IU/mL	4 mL clot-activator tube	As needed	Automated	Elevated ALP: skeletal disease, extrahepatic or intrahepatic biliary obstruction causing cholestasis	Ingestion of vitamin D, failure to analyze within 4 hours, drugs, pregnancy, age, and sex can affect results	N/A
	Gamma glutamyl transferase (GGT)	Assess liver function and to detect alcohol ingestion	• Men (> 16 years): 6–38 U/L • Women (16–45 years): 4–27 U/L • Women (>45 years): 6–37 U/L • Children (<16 years): 3–30 U/L	4 mL tube without additives	As needed	Automated	Elevated GGT: acute hepatic disease, alcohol ingestion, obstructive jaundice, acute pancreatitis, renal disease, and prostatic metastasis	N/A	N/A

Table 6-1: Overview of Urinalysis, Fluids, Chemistry, and Hematology Lab Tests *(continued)*

Chemistry									
General Category	Laboratory Test	Indications	Results	Specimen	Frequency	Test Type	Interpretation	Considerations for Test	Key Points
Liver function *(continued)*	Aspartate aminotransferase	Aids in diagnosing acute hepatic and myocardial infarction (MI)	8–46 U/L	4 mL clot-activator tube	As needed	Automated	• Levels >20 times normal: acute viral hepatitis, severe skeletal trauma, extensive surgery, drug-induced hepatic injury, or severe passive liver congestion • Level 10–20 times normal: severe MI, severe infectious mononucleosis, or alcoholic cirrhosis • Levels 5–10 times normal: dermatomyositis, Duchenne muscular dystrophy, or chronic hepatitis • Levels 2–5 times normal: hemolytic anemia, metastatic hepatic tumors, acute pancreatitis, pulmonary emboli, delirium tremens, or fatty liver	Various drugs such as opioids, large doses of acetaminophen, or vitamin A (not inclusive list) can affect results	N/A
Thyroid function	Triiodothyronine (T_3) uptake	Used for diagnosis of hypothyroidism and hyperthyroidism when thyroxine-binding globulin (TBG) is normal	25%–35%	7 mL clot-activator tube	As needed	Automated	• Hyperthyroidism: elevated T_3 uptake percentage when T_4 levels are high • Hypothyroidism: low T_3 uptake percentage with low T_4 levels	Radioisotope scan, anabolic steroids, heparin, hormonal contraceptives are examples of interfering factors	N/A

Table 6-1: Overview of Urinalysis, Fluids, Chemistry, and Hematology Lab Tests *(continued)*

Chemistry									
General Category	Laboratory Test	Indications	Results	Specimen	Frequency	Test Type	Interpretation	Considerations for Test	Key Points
Thyroid function *(continued)*	Free thyroxine (FT_4) and free triiodothyronine (FT_3)	Best indicator of thyroid function	• FT_4: 0.9–2.3 ng/dL • FT_3: 0.2–0.6 ng/dL (vary by laboratory)	8 mL clot-activator tube	As needed	Automated	• Elevated FT_4 and FT_3: hyperthyroidism unless thyroid hormone is present • Elevated FT_3 with normal or low FT_4: T_3 toxicosis (variation of hyperthyroidism) • Low FT_4: hypothyroidism except in patients receiving replacement therapy with T_3	Rarely used because of the cost and difficulty of the test; usually useful in the 5% of patients where total T_3 and T_4 failure to diagnose	N/A
	Thyroxine (T4) total	Evaluate thyroid function and monitor a patient's response to antithyroid medication	5–13.5 µg/dL	7 mL clot-activator tube	As needed	Automated	• Hyperthyroidism: elevated T_3 uptake percentage when T_4 levels are high • Hypothyroidism: low T_3 uptake percentage with low T_4 levels	Hereditary factors, hepatic disease, protein wasting disease, androgens, estrogens, methadone, free fatty acids, heparin, iodides, lithium, and other drugs (not inclusive list) can interfere with the test	N/A
	Thyroid-stimulating hormone (TSH)	Determines primary versus secondary hypothyroidism and monitors therapy	Undetectable: 15 µIU/mL	5 mL clot-activator tube	As needed	Automated	• Levels >20 µIU/mL: primary hypothyroidism or anemic goiter • Low levels or undetectable: normal or occasionally secondary hypothyroidism • Also hyperthyroidism (Graves disease) when there is hypersecretion of thyroid hormone (verified by TRH test)	Aspirin, steroids, thyroid hormones are interfering factors	N/A

Table 6-1: Overview of Urinalysis, Fluids, Chemistry, and Hematology Lab Tests *(continued)*

Chemistry									
General Category	Laboratory Test	Indications	Results	Specimen	Frequency	Test Type	Interpretation	Considerations for Test	Key Points
Thyroid function *(continued)*	Thyrotropin-releasing hormone (TRH)	Diagnostic for Graves disease	N/A	Requires injection of synthetic TRH by IV and then drawn 5, 10, 15, 20, and 60 minutes after injection	As needed	Automated	• Normal functioning pituitary: TSH has a sudden spike from baseline TSH after administration of TRH • Pituitary failure: TSH fails to rise or remains undetectable	N/A	N/A
	Calcium	Aids in evaluating endocrine function, and acid-base balance; monitored treatment of calcium deficiency, renal failure or transplant, malignancies, cardiac disease, and skeletal disorders	• Adults: 8.2–10.2 mg/dL • Children: 8.6–11.2 mg/dL Ionized 4.65–5.28 mg/dL	3–4 mL clot-activator tube	As needed	Automated	• Elevated results: Paget disease of the bone, metastatic carcinoma, multiple fractures, and prolonged immobilization • Decreased levels: renal failure, acute pancreatitis, peritonitis, and Cushing syndrome	Usually performed in conjunction with urine calcium and phosphate	N/A
	Iron	Used to estimate total iron storage, identify types of anemia, evaluate nutritional status, or diagnose hemochromatosis	• Men: 60–170 µg/dL • Women: 50–130 µg/dL	4.5 mL clot-activator tube	As needed	Automated	• Decreased iron levels occur in deficiency or in the presence of chronic inflammation • Iron overload may not alter serum levels until relatively late	Drugs such as chloramphenicol or contraceptives and iron supplements may affect iron test results	N/A
Diabetic testing	Fasting blood glucose (FBG); fasting blood sugar (FBS); fasting plasma glucose (FPG)	Screen for diabetes	• FPG adult: ≤110 mg/dL • Fasting children (2–18 years): 60–100 mg/dL • Fasting children (0–2 years): 60–110 mg/dL • Premature infants: 40–65 mg/dL	Serum if off red cells within 1 hour or gray top tube with sodium fluoride is acceptable for 24 hours	In morning for screening; as needed for self-monitoring	Automated test or portable for self-monitoring	• Elevated blood glucose: diabetes, Cushing disease, pituitary adenoma, and acute emotional or physical stress • Decreased blood plasma glucose: pancreatic islet cell carcinoma, liver damage, enzyme-deficiency diseases, and insulin overdose	Steroids, obesity, surgical procedures, IV glucose, heavy smoking, high hematocrit, intense exercise, overdose of some medications can affect glucose	N/A

Table 6-1: Overview of Urinalysis, Fluids, Chemistry, and Hematology Lab Tests *(continued)*

Chemistry

General Category	Laboratory Test	Indications	Results	Specimen	Frequency	Test Type	Interpretation	Considerations for Test	Key Points
Diabetic testing *(continued)*	Hemoglobin A1C	Useful in evaluating diabetic treatment	5.0%–7.0%	5 mL tube with EDTA anticoagulant	Every 3 months	Automated	Can be seen decreased in hemolytic anemia, chronic blood loss, pregnancy, and chronic renal failure	Presence of hemoglobin F, H, S, C, E, D, G can affect results	N/A
	Gestational diabetes mellitus	Test for glucose intolerance during pregnancy	130–140 mg/dL	5 mL with sodium fluoride additive; patient must be fasting	First prenatal visit and then at 24 to 28 weeks	Automated	If abnormal, a follow-up with a 3-hour glucose tolerance test should be performed	N/A	N/A
Arterial blood gas	Arterial oxygen (PaO_2)	Evaluate efficiency of pulmonary gas exchange, used for assessing ventilatory control system, acid-base level of the blood, and to monitor respiratory therapy	80–100 mm Hg	Heparinized blood gas syringe, eliminate air, and place on ice	As needed	Automated	• Low PaO_2, O_2CT, and SaO_2 levels with high $PaCO_2$: impaired respiratory function (respiratory muscle weakness, paralysis, respiratory center inhibition, airway obstruction [i.e., mucous plugs, or tumor]) • Low PaO_2, O_2CT, SaO_2 with normal $PaCO_2$: pneumothorax, interstitial fibrosis, or arteriovenous shunt that permits blood to bypass the lungs	Fever, exposing sample to air, and not drawing an arterial sample can interfere with results	• Used as part of the definition for PNU1, PNU2, and PNU3 in the NHSN definition • The PaO_2 is utilized in the worsening gas exchange ratio (PaO_2/FiO_2 ≤240)

Table 6-1: Overview of Urinalysis, Fluids, Chemistry, and Hematology Lab Tests (*continued*)

Chemistry									
General Category	Laboratory Test	Indications	Results	Specimen	Frequency	Test Type	Interpretation	Considerations for Test	Key Points
Arterial blood gas (*continued*)	Arterial carbon dioxide ($PaCO_2$)	Evaluate efficiency of pulmonary gas exchange, used for assessing ventilatory control system, acid-base level of the blood, and to monitor respiratory therapy	35–45 mm Hg	Heparinized blood gas syringe, eliminate air, and place on ice	As needed	Automated	• Low PaO_2, O_2CT, and SaO_2 levels with high $PaCO_2$: impaired respiratory function (respiratory muscle weakness, paralysis, respiratory center inhibition, airway obstruction [i.e., mucous plugs, or tumor]) • Low PaO_2, O_2CT, SaO_2 with normal $PaCO_2$: pneumothorax, interstitial fibrosis, or arteriovenous shunt that permits blood to bypass the lungs	Fever, exposing sample to air, not drawing an arterial sample, and certain drugs such as hydrocortisone, prednisone, nitrofurantoin, and tetracycline can affect test	N/A
	pH	Used to evaluate acid-base level of the blood and associated disorders	7.35–7.45	Heparinized blood gas syringe, eliminate air, and place on ice	As needed	Automated	• pH is used in conjunction with other arterial blood gas components ($PaCO_2$ and HCO_3) to determine if the patient is in metabolic acidosis/alkalosis and respiratory acidosis/alkalosis • Please see HCO_3 for further explanation	N/A	N/A

Table 6-1: Overview of Urinalysis, Fluids, Chemistry, and Hematology Lab Tests *(continued)*

Chemistry									
General Category	Laboratory Test	Indications	Results	Specimen	Frequency	Test Type	Interpretation	Considerations for Test	Key Points
Arterial blood gas *(continued)*	Oxygen content (O_2CT)	Evaluate efficiency of pulmonary gas exchange, used for assessing ventilatory control system, acid-base level of the blood, and to monitor respiratory therapy	15%–23%	Heparinized blood gas syringe, eliminate air, and place on ice	As needed	Automated	• Low PaO_2, O_2CT, and SaO_2 levels with high $PaCO_2$: impaired respiratory function (respiratory muscle weakness, paralysis, respiratory center inhibition, airway obstruction [i.e., mucous plugs, or tumor]) • Low PaO_2, O_2CT, SaO_2 with normal $PaCO_2$: pneumothorax, interstitial fibrosis, or arteriovenous shunt that permits blood to bypass the lungs • Low O_2CT with normal PaO_2, SaO_2, and maybe $PaCO_2$: severe anemia, decreased blood volume, and the ability to carry hemoglobin-oxygen is decreased	N/A	N/A
	Arterial oxygen saturation (SaO_2)	Evaluate efficiency of pulmonary gas exchange, used for assessing ventilatory control system, acid-base level of the blood, and to monitor respiratory therapy	94%–100%	Heparinized blood gas syringe, eliminate air, and place on ice	As needed	Automated	• Low PaO_2, O_2CT, and SaO_2 levels with high $PaCO_2$: impaired respiratory function (respiratory muscle weakness, paralysis, respiratory center inhibition, airway obstruction [i.e., mucous plugs, or tumor]) • Low PaO_2, O_2CT, SaO_2 with normal $PaCO_2$: pneumothorax, interstitial fibrosis, or arteriovenous shunt that permits blood to bypass the lungs	N/A	N/A

Table 6-1: Overview of Urinalysis, Fluids, Chemistry, and Hematology Lab Tests *(continued)*

Chemistry									
General Category	Laboratory Test	Indications	Results	Specimen	Frequency	Test Type	Interpretation	Considerations for Test	Key Points
Arterial blood gas *(continued)*	Bicarbonate (HCO_3^-)	Used to evaluate acid-base level of the blood and associated disorders	22–25 mEq/L	Heparinized blood gas syringe, eliminate air, and place on ice	As needed	Automated	• Low HCO_3^- in association with pH, SI, and $PaCO_2$: occurs in respiratory or metabolic acidosis • Respiratory acidosis: occurs in CNS depression, obesity, and asphyxia • Metabolic acidosis: excessive production of organic acids due to hepatic disease and endocrine disorders • High HCO_3^- in association with pH, SI, $PaCO_2$: occurs in respiratory or metabolic alkalosis • Respiratory alkalosis: improper vent setting, Gram-negative bacteremia, and chronic renal failure • Metabolic alkalosis: loss of acid due to vomiting or gastric suctioning, steroid overdose, and excessive alkali ingestion	N/A	N/A

Table 6-1: Overview of Urinalysis, Fluids, Chemistry, and Hematology Lab Tests *(continued)*

Hematology									
General Category	Laboratory Test	Indications	Results	Specimen	Frequency	Test Type	Interpretation	Considerations for Test	Key Points
Hematology	WBC count	Leukocytes fight infection and protect the body; clinicians use the WBC count to determine the severity of a disease based on the type of WBCs seen and how it correlates with clinical condition	• Adults: 4.5–10.5 × 103 cells/mm^3 C • Children 0–2 weeks: 9.0–30.0 × 103 cells/mm^3 • Children 2–8 weeks: 5.0–21.0 × 103 cells/mm^3 • Children 2 months to 6 years: 5.0–19.0 × 103 cells/ mm^3 • Children 6–18 years: 4.8–10.8 × 103 cells/mm^3	5 mL EDTA (lavender topped tube) of whole blood	As needed	Hemogram and complete blood count	• Leukocytosis (>11,000/mm^3): can occur in acute infection and the amount of WBC depends on the severity of the infection, patient's resistance, age, and immunity; can also occur in various other diseases such as leukemia, hemorrhage, and polycythemia vera; nonclinical causes are steroid therapy, sunlight, ultraviolet irradiation, and nausea • Leukopenia (<4,000/mm^3): can occur in viral or overwhelming bacterial infections; can also be caused by various cancers, and chemicals	Time, age, exercise, pain, temperature, and anesthesia can affect the WBC count	• Part of the PNU1, and PNU2 NHSN definition for pneumonia (<4,000 WBC/mm^3 or ≥12,000 WBC/mm^3) • For infants (≤ 1 year old), leukocytosis for PNU definition is defined as ≥15,000 WBC/mm^3 with a left shift (≥10% band forms) • For children >1 or ≤12 leukocytosis is defined as ≥15,000 WBC/mm^3 • The IP can use elevated WBC when evaluating bloodstream infections • Along with other signs and symptoms, it can be used as a tool to determine when the infection began

Table 6-1: Overview of Urinalysis, Fluids, Chemistry, and Hematology Lab Tests *(continued)*

Hematology									
General Category	Laboratory Test	Indications	Results	Specimen	Frequency	Test Type	Interpretation	Considerations for Test	Key Points
Hematology *(continued)*	RBC count	Determines the number of erythrocytes in a blood sample which is measure of the body's ability to carry oxygen	• Varied by age (most common) • Men: 4.2–5.4 × 106/mm³ • Women: 3.6–5.0 × 106/mm³	5 mL EDTA (lavender topped tube) of whole blood	As needed	Hemogram and complete blood count	• Decreased RBC count: can occur in various types of anemia, hemorrhage, myeloma, rheumatic fever, and subacute endocarditis or chronic infection • Increased RBC count: primary, secondary, and relative erythrocytosis	Posture, exercise, age, altitude, pregnancy, and many types of drugs can interfere with RBC count	N/A
	Hemoglobin	Used to evaluate severity of anemia and then how it responds to treatment	• Varied by age (most common) • Men: 14.0–17.4 g/dL • Women: 12.0–16.0 g/dL	5 mL EDTA (lavender topped tube) of whole blood	As needed	Hemogram and complete blood count	• Decreased: iron deficiency, liver disease, hemorrhage, hemolytic anemia, and various systemic diseases • Increased: COPD, CHF, polycythemia vera, and hemoglobin variants (i.e., sickle cell)	High altitude, excessive fluid intake, age, pregnancy, and many types of drugs can interfere with hemoglobin	Hemoglobin must be used in conjunction with the RBC count and hematocrit when evaluating anemia
	Hematocrit	Important measurement in the determination of anemia or polycythemia (volume of packed RBCs to whole blood)	• Varied by age (most common) • Men: 42%–52% • Women: 36%–48%	5 mL EDTA (lavender topped tube) of whole blood	As needed	Hemogram and complete blood count	• Decreased: indicator of anemia (HCT <30%) • Increased: occurs in erythrocytosis, polycythemia vera, or shock	Age, sex, and physiologic hydremia of pregnancy can affect hematocrit	N/A

Table 6-1: Overview of Urinalysis, Fluids, Chemistry, and Hematology Lab Tests *(continued)*

Hematology									
General Category	Laboratory Test	Indications	Results	Specimen	Frequency	Test Type	Interpretation	Considerations for Test	Key Points
Hematology *(continued)*	Mean corpuscular volume (MCV)	Cell volume is the best indicator for the type of anemia	82–98 fL (higher in infants and the elderly)	5 mL EDTA (lavender topped tube) of whole blood	As needed	Complete blood count	• MCV 50–82 fL: seen in disorders of iron metabolism, porphyrin and heme synthesis, and disorders of globin synthesis • MCV 82–98 fL: classifies normocytic normochromic anemias (both with appropriate and impaired bone marrow response) • MCV 100–150 fL: classifies macrocytic anemias (cobalamin, B12, and folate deficiencies)	Increased reticulocytes, leukocytosis, hyperglycemia, and cold agglutinins affect MCV	N/A
	Mean corpuscular hemoglobin (MCH)	Valuable in diagnosing severely anemic patients	24–34 pg/cell (can be higher in infants and newborns)	5 mL EDTA (lavender topped tube) of whole blood	As needed	Complete blood count	• Increased MCH: associated with macrocytic anemia • Decreased MCH: associated with microcytic anemia	High WBC counts, hyperlipidemia, and high heparin concentrations falsely elevate MCH	N/A
	Mean corpuscular hemoglobin concentration (MCHC)	Valuable in monitoring effectiveness of anemia therapy; this is a calculated value from Hb and HCT	32–36 g/dL	5 mL EDTA (lavender topped tube) of whole blood	As needed	Complete blood count	• Decreased MCHC: the unit volume of RBCs have less hemoglobin (Hgb) than normal which can occur in iron deficiency, some anemias, and thalassemia • Increased MCHC: occurs in spherocytosis which is hereditary or may be seen in newborns and infants	High values are found in newborns and infants; levels may increase due to leukemia, cold agglutinins, or a high concentration of heparin	N/A

Table 6-1: Overview of Urinalysis, Fluids, Chemistry, and Hematology Lab Tests *(continued)*

Hematology									
General Category	Laboratory Test	Indications	Results	Specimen	Frequency	Test Type	Interpretation	Considerations for Test	Key Points
Hematology *(continued)*	Platelet count	Used for evaluating bleeding disorders and for monitoring any disease course associated with the bone marrow	• Adults: 140–00 × 103/mm³ • Children: 150–450 × 103/mm³	5 mL EDTA (lavender topped tube) of whole blood	As needed	• Hemogram and complete blood count • Also seen on manual differential if needed	• Elevated platelets: seen in various disorders such as acute infections, inflammatory diseases, chronic pancreatitis, tuberculosis, inflammatory bowel disease, and renal failure • Decreased platelets: seen in viral, bacterial, and rickettsial infections, CHF, HIV, eclampsia, and renal insufficiency	A clotted blood specimen, high altitudes, strenuous exercise, excitement, oral contraception, premenstrual and postpartum effects can all affect platelets	N/A
	RBC distribution width (RDW)	Helps with diagnosing hematologic disorders and monitoring therapy via the degree of anisocytosis (abnormal variation in RBC size)	11.5–14.5 coefficient of variation (CV) of red cell size	5 mL EDTA (lavender topped tube) of whole blood	As needed	Complete blood count	• With MCV, it can separate various types of anemia • Increased RDW: found in iron deficiency, pernicious anemia, and hemolytic anemia • Normal RDW: seen in chronic disease, acute blood lost, and sickle cell disease • There are no causes of decreased RDW	Alcohol and cold agglutinins can interfere with RDW	N/A
	Mean platelet volume (MPV)	Used for differential diagnosis of thrombocytopenia	Adults and children : 7.4–10.4 μm³	5 mL EDTA (lavender topped tube) of whole blood	As needed	Complete blood count	• Elevated MPV: seen in thrombocytopenia caused by sepsis, prosthetic heart valve, massive hemorrhage, and myelogenous leukemia • Decreased MPV: seen with Wiskott-Aldrich syndrome	N/A	N/A

Table 6-1: Overview of Urinalysis, Fluids, Chemistry, and Hematology Lab Tests *(continued)*

Hematology									
General Category	Laboratory Test	Indications	Results	Specimen	Frequency	Test Type	Interpretation	Considerations for Test	Key Points
Hematology *(continued)*	Segmented neutrophils (polymorphonuclear neutrophils, PMNs, polys)	PMNs react to inflammation, primary defense against microbial invasion	• Absolute counts: 3,000-7,000/mm^3 • Black adults: 1.2–6.6 × 109/L • Differential: 50% of total WBC 0%–3% of total neutrophils are band cells	5 mL EDTA (lavender topped tube) of whole blood	As needed	Manual differential	• Neutrophilia (increased neutrophil count: 8,000/mm^3 or for African Americans 7,000/mm^3): seen with inflammation, bacterial infections, and early stages of viral infections • A shift to the left or increase in bands is a sign of infections • If leukocytosis is present, the prognosis of recovery is good; if not, prognosis is the opposite • Neutropenia (decrease in neutrophils: <1,800/mm^3 and in African Americans <1,000/mm^3): occurs in overwhelming bacterial infections, viral infections such as hepatitis, influenza, and hematopoietic disease	Physiologic conditions (stress, shock, anger, joy, etc.), labor, steroid administration, exposure to extreme heat or cold, age, resistance can all affect neutrophil counts	• PNU3 NHSN definition to determine immunocompromised patients, the ANC must be <500/mm^3 • For children ≤1 leukocytosis is defined in the PNU definition as 15,000 WBC/mm^3 with a left shift (≥10% band forms)

Table 6-1: Overview of Urinalysis, Fluids, Chemistry, and Hematology Lab Tests *(continued)*

Hematology									
General Category	Laboratory Test	Indications	Results	Specimen	Frequency	Test Type	Interpretation	Considerations for Test	Key Points
Hematology *(continued)*	Eosinophils	Responds to allergic and parasitic diseases; used to diagnose allergic infections, and assess parasitic infestations	• Absolute count: 0–0.7 × 109/L • Differential: 0%–3% of total WBC	5 mL EDTA (lavender topped tube) of whole blood	As needed	Manual differential	• Eosinophilia (increased: >500 cells/mm^3): seen in allergies, hay fever, chronic skin disease, parasitic disease, and trichinosis tapeworm, Crohn disease, poisons, and some immunodeficiency disorders • Eosinopenia (decreased): stems from an increase in adrenal steroid production which results from Cushing syndrome, use of certain drugs (ACTH, epinephrine), and acute bacterial infections with a marked shift to the left	• Eosinophil counts vary by the time of day so when repeating tests, they should be done at the same time every day • Other interfering factors are burns, electroshock, and postoperative states	N/A

Table 6-1: Overview of Urinalysis, Fluids, Chemistry, and Hematology Lab Tests *(continued)*

Hematology									
General Category	Laboratory Test	Indications	Results	Specimen	Frequency	Test Type	Interpretation	Considerations for Test	Key Points
Hematology *(continued)*	Basophils	Used to study chronic inflammation	• Absolute count: 15–50/mm^3 • Differential: 0%–1.0% of total WBC	5 mL EDTA (lavender topped tube) of whole blood	As needed	Manual differential	• Basophilia (increased: >50/mm^3): seen in granulocytic or acute basophilic leukemia, Hodgkin disease, and sometimes in inflammation, allergy, or infections from tuberculosis (TB), smallpox, chickenpox, or influenza • Basopenia (decreased: <20/mm^3): seen in acute phase of infection, stress reactions, prolonged steroid or chemotherapy, and acute rheumatic fever in children • If tissue mast cells are seen (tissue basophils), it can be related to rheumatoid arthritis, anaphylactic shock, some types of cancer, and chronic or renal disease	Some drugs can affect the basophilic count	N/A

Table 6-1: Overview of Urinalysis, Fluids, Chemistry, and Hematology Lab Tests *(continued)*

Hematology									
General Category	Laboratory Test	Indications	Results	Specimen	Frequency	Test Type	Interpretation	Considerations for Test	Key Points
Hematology *(continued)*	Monocytes	Can indicate the recovery phase of acute infection	• Absolute count: 100–200/mm^3 • Differential: 3%–7% of total WBC	5 mL EDTA (lavender topped tube) of whole blood	As needed	Manual differential	• Monocytosis (increase: >500 cells/mm^3): seen in bacterial infections, TB, subacute bacterial endocarditis, syphilis, recovery state of neutropenia (favorable sign), some parasites, and surgical trauma • In severe infections, phagocytic monocytes (macrophages) can be seen • Decreased monocyte count (<100 cells/mm^3): seen in HIV, aplastic anemia, or an overwhelming infection that causes neutropenia	Some drugs can affect the basophilic count	N/A

Table 6-1: Overview of Urinalysis, Fluids, Chemistry, and Hematology Lab Tests *(continued)*

Hematology									
General Category	Laboratory Test	Indications	Results	Specimen	Frequency	Test Type	Interpretation	Considerations for Test	Key Points
Hematology *(continued)*	Lymphocytes	Lymphocytes are an important part of the immune response and can be prominent in viral infections	• Absolute count: 1,500–4,000 cells/mm^3 • Differential: 25%–40% of total WBC	5 mL EDTA (lavender topped tube) of whole blood	As needed	Manual differential	• Lymphocytosis (increased: >4,000 cells/mm^3 in adults, >7,200 cells/mm^3 in children and >9,000 cells/mm^3 in infants): seen in infectious mononucleosis, different types of leukemia, viral infections of the upper respiratory tract, CMV, measles, mumps, chickenpox, and viral hepatitis • Lymphopenia (decreased: <1,000 cells/mm^3 in adults, <2,500 in children): occurs from chemotherapy, steroids, some immune disorders, CHF, and miliary tuberculosis	Drugs, exercise, emotional stress, some pediatric lymphocytosis can affect lymphocyte presence	N/A
	CD4 count	Master immune cells; the presence or absence can indicate the body's ability to fight off infection	CD4/CD8 ratio: >1.0	5 mL EDTA (lavender topped tube) of whole blood	As needed	Flow cytometry	• Decreased CD4: present in immune dysfunction (i.e., HIV) and acute minor viral infections • Increased CD4: can be from drug or natural variation • Formula: CD4 count: total WBC × lymphocytes (%) × lymphocytes (%) stained with CD4	N/A	Part of PNU3 NHSN definition to determine immunocompromised patients, the CD4 count must be <200

Table 6-1: Overview of Urinalysis, Fluids, Chemistry, and Hematology Lab Tests *(continued)*

Hematology									
General Category	Laboratory Test	Indications	Results	Specimen	Frequency	Test Type	Interpretation	Considerations for Test	Key Points
Hematology *(continued)*	Stained red cell examination	Useful in examining blood disorders	• Normal size: 7–8 μm • Color: normochromic • Shape: biconcave disk • Structure: normocytes or erythrocytes (anucleated cells)	5 mL EDTA (lavender topped tube) of whole blood	As needed	Manual differential	• Various cells can be seen and will help diagnose blood disorders • For example, the presence of schistocytes can be a result of an artificial heart valve, toxins, renal graft reject, or DIC	N/A	N/A
	Reticulocyte count	Used to differentiate anemia caused by bone marrow failure versus hemorrhage; also used to evaluate therapy and the effects of radioactive substances on exposed workers	• Adults: 0.5%–1.5% of total erythrocytes • Newborns: 3%–6% of total erythrocytes	5 mL EDTA (lavender topped tube) of whole blood	As needed	Stain with a supravital stain	• Increased reticulocyte count: occurs when the bone marrow is producing erythrocytes to replace what has been lost such as hemolytic anemia and hemorrhage • Decreased reticulocyte count: occurs when the bone marrow is not producing enough erythrocytes such as aplastic anemia, untreated pernicious anemia, and radiation therapy	N/A	N/A
	Erythrocyte sedimentation rate (ESR)	Useful in diagnosis of some types of arthritis (rheumatoid), monitoring progression of inflammatory diseases, and treatment	• Using Westergren's method: Men: 0–15 mm/hour Women: 0–20 mm/hour Newborn: 0–2 mm/hour Children: 0–10 mm/hour	5 mL EDTA (lavender topped tube) of whole blood	As needed	Westergren's method	• Increased ESR: seen in all collagen disease, inflammatory diseases, carcinoma, toxemia, and infections (pneumonia, syphilis, and TB) • Normal ESR: can be seen in sickle cell, CHF, uncomplicated viral disease, and infectious mononucleosis	Refrigerated blood, menstruation, young children, high blood sugar, certain drugs, high WBCs can all interfere with test	N/A

Table 6-1: Overview of Urinalysis, Fluids, Chemistry, and Hematology Lab Tests *(continued)*

Hematology									
General Category	Laboratory Test	Indications	Results	Specimen	Frequency	Test Type	Interpretation	Considerations for Test	Key Points
Hematology *(continued)*	G6PD	Aids in testing for G6PD deficiency	• G6PD screen: detected • Adults: 8.6–18.6 U/g Hb • Children: 6.4–15.6 U/g Hb • Newborns have values up to 50% higher than adults	5 mL of whole blood in two lavender topped tubes (EDTA or heparin antico-agulant) and place on ice	As needed	G6PD	• Decreased G6PD: seen in G6PD defi-ciency, congenital nonsperocytic ane-mia, nonimmunolog-ic hemolytic disease of the newborn • Elevated G6PD: seen in untreated pernicious anemia, thrombocytopenia purpura, hyperthy-roidism, and viral hepatitis	Marked reticulocy-tosis and a recent episode of anemia can affect G6PD	N/A
Coagulation	Bleeding time	Diagnosis of von Willebrand disease	3–10 minutes	Performed on patient using blood pressure cuff, stopwatch, and a 4 x 4-inch filter paper	As needed	Ivym	Prolonged bleeding time occurs when platelets are de-creased or abnormal (i.e., thrombocytope-nia, advanced renal failure, DIC, scurvy are some examples)	Excessive alcohol consumption, inges-tion of aspirin up to 5 days before test, extreme hot and cold, and edema of patient's hands can affect the test	N/A
	Thrombin time (TT); thrombin clotting time (TCT)	Detects stage III fibrinogen de-fects, DIC, hypo-fibrinogenemia, and monitoring streptokinase therapy	7.0–12.0 sec-onds	Two tube specimen collected in sodium citrate and placed on ice (or frozen if not performed within 2 hours)	As needed	TT or TCT	• Prolonged TT: seen in DIC, hypofibri-nogenemia, multiple myeloma, severe liver disease, and uremia • Shortened TT: Oc-curs in hyperfibrino-genemia and elevated HCT (>55%)	Heparin, plasmino-gen activator therapy, and some drugs affect outcome	N/A
	Partial throm-boplastin time (PTT) or acti-vated partial thromboplastin time (APTT)	• PTT screens for coagulation disorders • APTT detects deficiencies in the coagula-tion system, detect incubating anticoagulants, and to monitor heparin therapy	• 21.0–35.0 seconds • Therapeutic ranges depend on the labora-tory	5 mL venous blood specimen collected in sodium citrate	As needed or for heparin therapy: baseline, 1 hour before next dose, and according to patient's bleed-ing status	PTT or APTT	• Prolonged APTT: seen with heparin or warfarin therapy, vitamin K deficiency, liver disease, and DIC • Shortened APTT: seen with extensive cancer (except liver), after acute hemor-rhage, and early stages of DIC	N/A	When APTT is performed with PT, the coagulation defect can be clarified in the clotting cascade

Table 6-1: Overview of Urinalysis, Fluids, Chemistry, and Hematology Lab Tests (*continued*)

Hematology									
General Category	Laboratory Test	Indications	Results	Specimen	Frequency	Test Type	Interpretation	Considerations for Test	Key Points
Coagulation (*continued*)	Prothrombin time (PT)	Used in diagnostic coagulation studies	• 11.0–13.0 seconds • Therapeutic ranges are based on surgery type or disease	5 mL venous blood specimen collected in sodium citrate	As needed or when evaluating therapy every day until therapeutic range is reached and then weekly to monthly for duration of therapy	PT	• Increased PT: can be caused by several conditions such as vitamin K deficiency, DIC, liver disease, and premature newborns • Unaffected PT: can be found in polycythemia vera, Tannin disease, hemophilia A, and platelet disorders	Digestion of green leafy vegetables, diarrhea, alcoholism, and some drugs can affect PT	N/A
	Coagulant factors (II–XII)	Used for investigation of inherited or acquired bleeding disorders	Depends on factor (please check with laboratory for reference)	5 mL venous blood specimen collected in sodium citrate, and placed on ice	As needed	Coagulant factor	• The deficiencies of each factor in the coagulation pathway can be associated with various deficiencies • For a comprehensive list, please see a reference manual	N/A	N/A
	Plasminogen (plasmin, fibrinolysin)	Used to determine plasminogen activity in persons with thrombosis or DIC	• Men: 76%–124% of normal for plasma • Women: 65%–153% of normal for plasma • Infants: 27%–59% of normal for plasma	• Two tube specimen collected in sodium citrate and placed on ice • Must be performed within 30 minutes after blood is drawn	As needed	Plasminogen	• Increased plasminogen: can be seen in the third trimester of pregnancy, or regular vigorous physical exercise • Decreased plasminogen: can be seen in DIC and systemic fibrinolysis, liver disease, and cirrhosis	Some drugs can affect outcomes	N/A
	Fibrinolysis (euglobulin lysis time; diluted whole blood clot lysis)	Evaluate fibrinolytic activity	• Euglobulin lysis: no lysis of plasma clot at 37°C in 60–120 minutes • Diluted whole blood clot lysis: no lysis of clot in 120 minutes at 37°C	• Two tube specimen collected in sodium citrate and placed on ice • Must be performed within 30 minutes after blood is drawn	As needed	Fibrinolysis	Increased fibrinolysis: can occur within 48 hours of surgery, prostate or pancreas cancer, liver disease, and cardiac surgery	Moderate exercise, increasing age, arterial blood, postmenopause, and a traumatic venipuncture are some interfering factors	N/A

Table 6-1: Overview of Urinalysis, Fluids, Chemistry, and Hematology Lab Tests *(continued)*

Hematology									
General Category	Laboratory Test	Indications	Results	Specimen	Frequency	Test Type	Interpretation	Considerations for Test	Key Points
Coagulation *(continued)*	Fibrin split products (FSP); fibrin degradation products (FDP)	Used to help diagnose DIC and other thromboembolic disorders	Negative is a 1:4 dilution	4.5 mL blood sample in a tube with an inhibitor of fibrinolysis and thrombin	As needed	FSP/FDP	High FSP/FDP: means the blood does not clot properly and can be seen in AMI, pulmonary embolism, carcinoma, primary fibrinolysis, and venous thrombosis	Heparin therapy, and presence of rheumatoid factor	N/A
	D-dimer	Used to help diagnose DIC, AMI, and to screen for venous thrombosis	<250 µg/L	5 mL blood collected in sodium citrate and aprotinin	As needed	D-dimer	Increased D-dimer: can be seen in DIC, deep vein thrombosis, renal or liver failure, pulmonary embolism, MI, malignancy, inflammation, and severe infection	Presence of rheumatoid factor, ovarian cancer, surgery, estrogen therapy, and pregnancy can affect the test	N/A

References

Allen K et al. *Lippincott Manual of Nursing Practice Series: Diagnostic Tests*. Philadelphia: Lippincott Williams & Wilkins, 2007.

Horan TC, Andrus M, Dudeck MA. CDC/NHSN surveillance definition of healthcare-associated infection and criteria for specific types of infections in the acute care setting. *Am J Infect Control* 2008;36(5):309–332.

Humes HD, Kelley WN. *Kelley's Textbook of Internal Medicine*, 4th ed. Philadelphia: Lippincott Williams & Wilkins, 2000.

Irwin RS, Rippe JM, Lisbon A, Heard SO. *Procedures, Techniques, and Minimally Invasive Monitoring in Intensive Care Medicine*, 4th ed. Philadelphia: Lippincott Williams & Wilkins, 2008.

Light RW. *Pleural Diseases*, 5th ed. Philadelphia: Lippincott Williams & Wilkins, 2007.

Fishman SM, Ballantyne JC, Rathmell JP. *Bonica's Management of Pain*, 4th ed. Philadelphia: Lippincott Williams & Wilkins, 2009.

Lotke PA. *Lippincott's Primary Care Orthopaedic*. Philadelphia: Lippincott Williams & Wilkins, 2008.

Weinstein S, Plumer LA. *Plumer's Principles & Practice of Intravenous Therapy*, 8th ed. Philadelphia: Lippincott Williams & Wilkins, 2007.

Chapter 7

Mycobacteriology

Carolyn Fiutem, MT(ASCP), CIC

Mycobacteria are ubiquitous in nature. Most can be found as free living organisms, while others act as obligate parasites. The *Mycobacterium* genus is comprised of rapid growers (grow in less than 7 days) and slow growers (take longer than 7 days to grow) which includes the *M. tuberculosis* complex.

Mycobacterial infections can affect any area of the body. They can cause acute or chronic infections, are difficult to diagnose, and problematic to treat. Mycobacteria cause infections such as leprosy (*Mycobacterium leprae*) and skin and soft tissue infection associated with fish tanks (*Mycobacterium marinum*). *Mycobacterium abscessus* is a rapid grower and often a water contaminant. It causes chronic lung disease, disseminated cutaneous disease in immunocompromised patients, and posttraumatic wound infections. *Mycobacterium chelonae*, also a rapid grower, is often found in water and sewage and will cause occasional opportunistic infections. *Mycobacterium fortuitum* is a rapid grower that can be found in localized skin infections, osteomyelitis, joint infections, and posttraumatic eye infections. *Mycobacterium kansasii* is a slow grower that is a water contaminant and may cause disease in patients with severely impaired cellular immunity.

The mycobacteria other than tuberculosis (MOTT) group can cause other pulmonary diseases. The most common is *Mycobacterium avium-intracellulare* complex, which can cause chronic lung infections in patients with compromised lungs. The MOTT group can also be a nuisance in the laboratory if specimens become contaminated with tap water or if procedural instruments, such as bronchoscopes, are improperly processed and contaminated with tap water.

The mycobacterial infection of the most significance to the infection preventionist is tuberculosis, which is caused by *Mycobacterium tuberculosis*. *M. tuberculosis* is one of several slow-growing mycobacteria in the *M. tuberculosis* complex. The *M. tuberculosis* complex is comprised of *M. tuberculosis, M. bovis, M. africanum,* and *M. microti*.

When testing specimen and isolates for mycobacteria, microbiologists must wear personal protective equipment and conduct tests in a special negative pressure room and under a biological cabinet, with laminar flow. Mycobacteria require special processing to eliminate other faster-growing bacteria, yeasts, or fungi that might be present in the specimen. Special media are used for culturing to meet the nutritional needs of the mycobacteria—this includes solid media, plates and tubes, and broth media. Because of the slower growth nature of this group and the need to know the infecting agent, rapid means to recover and identify this group are necessary. There are a wide variety of techniques available, depending on the specific need.

The following table is a summary of testing methodologies for mycobacteria, including their advantages and disadvantages, appropriate use, and test limitations. It is intended to help the infection preventionist make educated recommendations pertaining to patient placement and exposure follow-up. Many of these procedures are performed by reference laboratories rather than in the hospitals. Some of the techniques are quite expensive to perform and are highly specialized, requiring additional knowledge to perform and interpret.

Table 7-1: Overview of Mycobacteria Testing Methodologies

Specimen Collection and Transport: When collecting and transporting specimens to laboratories for testing, consult the lab for collection and transport instructions and adhere to following regulations:

• Private courier: IATA Packaging Instructions 602 for pure culture isolates; IATA Packaging Instructions 650 for clinical specimens

• US Postal Service: If sending either type of specimen, see USPS Packaging Instruction 6D at http://pe.usps.com/text/pub52/pub52apxc_021.htm

General category	Laboratory Test	Indications	Specific Microbes	Specimen	Frequency	Test Type	Interpretation	Advantages/ Disadvantages	Sample Transport	Key Points
Microscopy	Acid-fast bacillus (AFB) smear	Diagnostic	*Mycobacterium tuberculosis* (MTB), mycobacteria other than tuberculosis (MOTT) speciated	• Respiratory • Gastric wash (usually pediatrics) • Body fluids • Cerebrospinal fluid (CSF) • Tissue • Urine • Aspirated pus • Blood • Bone marrow • Less optimal raw specimens: stool, swabs	• Respiratory/gastric wash: early morning specimen daily times three • Others: as specimen available	Smear: direct smear and concentrated smear	AFB seen or no AFB seen	• Rapid test for which a positive test would warrant placing patients into airborne precautions without waiting for culture results • Although positive tests can be definitive for mycobacterial disease, they cannot be considered for any case or used as a stand-alone test • Test sensitivity can be as low as 60% because ~ 10,000 organisms/mL of specimen is needed for a visibly positive smear	• Respiratory and urine: refrigerate, transport cold; preferably within one hour of collection • Bone marrow and blood: collect in a tube with SPS anticoagulant • Stool: collect no more than 10 mL in a 50-mL polypropylene tube and securely tighten the lid • Swabs: place in 10 mls of 7H9 broth or sterile saline in a 50 ml conical tube; specimen does not offer much sensitivity due to minimal specimen • All others: transport to lab immediately	Sensitivity can be dependent on whether it is performed on a direct specimen smear or a concentrated specimen smear, the number of AFB in the specimen, and the experience of medical technologist/ microscopist

Table 7-1: Overview of Mycobacteria Testing Methodologies (continued)

General category	Laboratory Test	Indications	Specific Microbes	Specimen	Frequency	Test Type	Interpretation	Advantages/ Disadvantages	Sample Transport	Key Points
Culture	AFB culture	Diagnostic	MTB, MOTT speciated	• Respiratory, including induced sputum • Gastric wash (usually pediatrics) • Body fluids • CSF • Tissue • Urine • Aspirated pus • Blood • Bone marrow • Less optimal raw specimens: stool - when contaminated food or milk questions exist, swabs	• Respiratory/gastric wash: early morning specimen daily times three • Others: as specimen available	Culture (solid media and liquid/broth media) and identification	• Growth of mycobacteria • Based on biochemical test results for identification on isolates or molecular testing on the isolate • Or no growth of mycobacteria after 6 or 8 weeks, depending on the individual laboratory protocols	• Depending on the organism and amount present, can take a few days to weeks to grow • Culture method has the advantage of allowing performance of susceptibility testing on the organism to better guide treatment modalities.	• Respiratory and urine: refrigerate, transport cold; swabs should be placed in 10 mL of 7H9 broth or sterile saline in a 50-mL conical tube. • Bone marrow and blood: collect in a tube with SPS anticoagulant • Stool: collect no more than 10 mL in a 50-mL polypropylene tube and securely tighten the lid • All others: transport to lab immediately	Recovery can be dependent on the quality of the specimen, processing of the specimen, and incubation conditions, as well as any treatment history of the patient as antibiotic damaged organisms can take longer to grow
Biochemical Phenotypic Method	Biochemical test	Diagnostic	MTB, MOTT speciated	Isolate: on solid media	Only needed on one of the isolates of a specimen	Identification from culture by phenotypic method	*Mycobacterium*	• Inexpensive but slow • Availability is lab dependent	Refer to specimen transport instructions at the beginning of this table	Methods used are laboratory dependent; consult with reference laboratory for methods and uses available
Advanced Biochemical	High Pressure Liquid Chromatography (HPLC) or Gas Liquid Chromatography (GLC)	Diagnostic	MTB, MOTT speciated	• Isolate on solid media • For HPLC, broth can also be used • For GLC, extracted cell lipids are tested	Only needed on one of the isolates of a specimen	Identification	*Mycobacterium*	Expensive but rapid; availability is lab dependent	Refer to specimen transport instructions at the beginning of this table	Methods used are laboratory dependent; consult with reference laboratory for methods and uses available

Table 7-1: Overview of Mycobacteria Testing Methodologies (*continued*)

General category	Laboratory Test	Indications	Specific Microbes	Specimen	Frequency	Test Type	Interpretation	Advantages/ Disadvantages	Sample Transport	Key Points
Susceptibility	AFB sensitivity test	Treatment guidance	MTB, MOTT speciated	Isolate: on solid media or in liquid/broth media	• Only need to perform on the isolate(s) from the first positive specimen • Testing on all initial positive specimens not necessary	Susceptibility	S = susceptible I = intermediate R = resistant MICs (mean inhibitory concentration) may accompany result to aid in treatment/ dosing determinations	Used to determine if isolate is multidrug resistant (MDR) or extra-multidrug resistant (XDR) to guide treatment modalities, isolation, and follow-up	Refer to specimen transport instructions at the beginning of this table	Can take time, depending on method used (liquid media: MIC vs. disk diffusion) and growth rate of the isolate (rapid grower vs. slow grower)
Molecular testing	DNA Probe and/ or RNA or mitochondrial probe	Diagnostic and/or treatment guidance	MTB, MOTT speciated	• Respiratory • Gastric wash (usually pediatrics) • Body fluids • CSF • Tissue • Urine • Aspirated pus • Blood • Bone marrow • Less optimal raw specimens: swabs, stool • Can also send isolate: on solid media or in liquid/broth media	• Only needed on one of the isolates of a specimen • Test specimen as available	Identification from positive culture	• *Mycobacterium* • May include susceptibility information	• Initial start-up is an investment • Commercially available and easy for staff to perform • Rapid • It must be emphasized that although positive results are most helpful for rapid positive diagnoses, smear negative specimens can frequently give falsely negative results due to the technical difficulty in releasing of adequate nucleic acids to meet the sensitivity requirements of current molecular tests • NOTE: the FDA and some manufacturers have recommended that negative molecular tests be confirmed subsequently by culture.	• Respiratory and urine: refrigerate, transport cold • Bone marrow and blood: collect in a tube with SPS anticoagulant • Stool: collect no more than 10 mL in a 50-mL polypropylene tube and securely tighten the lid • Swabs: place in 10 mls of 7H9 broth or sterile saline in a 50 ml conical tube. • All others: transport to lab immediately; if sending to an outside lab, refer to specimen transport instructions at the beginning of this table	Determine lab needs to select most appropriate commercially available test; some commercially available test can be rapid and easy for staff to perform.

Table 7-1: Overview of Mycobacteria Testing Methodologies *(continued)*

General category	Laboratory Test	Indications	Specific Microbes	Specimen	Frequency	Test Type	Interpretation	Advantages/ Disadvantages	Sample Transport	Key Points
Molecular testing for identification	DNA sequencing, also known as gene sequencing, complete genome sequencing or partial genome sequencing of 16S rRNA, 23S rRNA, *ITS1* gene, *Nsp65* gene, *rpoB* gene, *gyrB* gene	Diagnostic	MTB, MOTT speciated	Isolate: on solid media or in liquid/broth media	Only needed on one of the isolates of a specimen	Identification from positive culture	*Mycobacterium*	• Expensive but rapid • Availability is lab dependent	Refer to specimen transport instructions at the beginning of this table	Methods used are laboratory dependent; consult with reference laboratory for methods and uses available
Molecular testing for identification	MIRU-VNTR typing	Strain typing, epidemiologic work-up	MTB	Isolate: on solid media	Only needed on one of the isolates of a specimen	Epidemiology from culture	MTB	• Expensive but rapid • Availability is lab dependent	Refer to specimen transport instructions at the beginning of this table	Methods used are laboratory dependent; consult with reference laboratory for methods and uses available
Molecular testing for identification	Nucleic acid amplification (NAA)	Diagnostic	MTB, MOTT speciated	• Respiratory • Gastric wash (usually peds) • Body fluids • CSF • Tissue • Urine • Aspirated pus • Blood • Bone marrow • Less optimal raw specimens: swabs, stool • Isolate: on solid media or in liquid/broth media	• Only needed on one specimen • Test specimen as available	Direct identification from specimen	*Mycobacterium*	• Expensive but rapid • Availability is lab dependent	Refer to specimen transport instructions at the beginning of this table	Methods used are laboratory dependent; consult with reference laboratory for methods and uses available

Table 7-1: Overview of Mycobacteria Testing Methodologies (continued)

General category	Laboratory Test	Indications	Specific Microbes	Specimen	Frequency	Test Type	Interpretation	Advantages/ Disadvantages	Sample Transport	Key Points
Molecular testing for detection of antimicrobial resistance	Line probe assay	Diagnostic and/or treatment guidance	MDR or XDR *M. tuberculosis* (Mtb)	• AFB smear positive sputum • Isolate: on solid media or in liquid/broth media	Only needed on one isolate	Susceptibility markers for Mtb complex and MDR-Mtb, to be used in high-risk populations	• Presence of *M. tuberculosis* complex • Probable MDR strain detected based on mutations detected	• Rapid detection of Mtb complex and MDR or XDR Mtb • Fairly significant preparations required • Prone to cross-contamination (false positive) • Prohibitively expensive in many areas where needed	Refer to specimen transport instructions at the beginning of this table	Lower sensitivity when used directly on sputum versus the isolate; consult reference laboratory on use guidance and markers available
Molecular testing for detection	Polymerase chain reaction (PCR)	Diagnostic	MTB, MOTT speciated	• Respiratory • Gastric wash (usually pediatrics) • Body fluids • CSF • Tissue • Urine • Aspirated pus • Blood • Bone marrow • Less optimal raw specimens: swabs, stool • Isolate: on solid media or in liquid/broth media	• Only needed on one specimen • Test specimen as available	Direct identification from specimen	*Mycobacterium*	• Initial start-up is an investment • Commercially available and easy for staff to perform • Rapid	• Respiratory and urine: refrigerate, transport cold; swabs should be placed in 10 mL of 7H9 broth or sterile saline in a 50-mL conical tube • Bone marrow and blood: collect in a tube with SPS anticoagulant • Stool: collect no more than 10 mL in a 50-mL polypropylene tube and securely tighten the lid • All others: transport to lab immediately; if sending to an outside lab, refer to specimen transport instructions at the beginning of this table	Determine lab needs to select most appropriate commercially available test

Table 7-1: Overview of Mycobacteria Testing Methodologies *(continued)*

General category	Laboratory Test	Indications	Specific Microbes	Specimen	Frequency	Test Type	Interpretation	Advantages/ Disadvantages	Sample Transport	Key Points
Molecular testing for strain typing	Pulse field gel electrophoresis (PFGE)	Strain typing, epidemiologic work-up	MTB, MOTT speciated	Isolate: on solid media or in liquid/broth media	Only needed on one of the isolates of a specimen	Epidemiology	*Mycobacterium*	• Expensive but rapid • Availability is lab dependent	Refer to specimen transport instructions at the beginning of this table	Methods used are laboratory dependent; consult with reference laboratory for methods and uses available
Molecular testing for strain typing	IS6110 restriction fragment length polymorphism (RFLP) typing	Strain typing, epidemiologic work-up	MTB	Isolate: on solid media or in liquid/broth media	Only needed on one of the isolates of a specimen	Epidemiology from culture	MTB	• Expensive but rapid • Availability is lab dependent	Refer to specimen transport instructions at the beginning of this table	Methods used are laboratory dependent; consult with reference laboratory for methods and uses available
Molecular testing for strain typing	Spacer oligotyping (spoligotyping)	Strain typing; epidemiologic work-up	MTB	Isolate: on solid media or in liquid/broth media	Only needed on one of the isolates of a specimen	Epidemiology from culture	MTB	• Expensive but rapid • Availability is lab dependent	Refer to specimen transport instructions at the beginning of this table	Methods used are laboratory dependent; consult with reference laboratory for methods and uses available

References

Garcia, LS, Isenberg HD. Mycobacteriology and Antimycobacterial Susceptibility Testing. In: Garcia LS, ed. *Clinical Microbiology Procedures Handbook*, 3rd ed. Washington, DC: American Society for Microbiology, 2010.

National Jewish Health. *Mycobacteriology (TB) laboratory: requisitions and specimen handling.* National Jewish Health: National Jewish Health Web site. 2011. Available at http://www.nationaljewish.org/research/diagnostics/adx/ labs/mycobacteriology/requisitions-and-specimen-handling. Accessed October 1, 2011.

Pfyffer GE, Palicova F. Mycobacterium: General Characteristics, Laboratory Detection, and Staining Procedures. In: Versalovic J, ed. *Manual of Clinical Microbiology*, 10th ed. Washington, DC: ASM, 2011.

Richter E, Brown-Elliott BA, Wallace RJ. Mycobacterium: Laboratory Characteristics of Slowly Growing Mycobacteria. In: Versalovic J, ed. *Manual of Clinical Microbiology*, 10th ed. Washington, DC: ASM, 2011.

Spellerberg B, Brandt C. Streptococcus. In: Versalovic J, ed. *Manual of Clinical Microbiology*, 10th ed. Washington, DC: ASM, 2011.

Woods GL, Lin SYG, Desmond EP. Susceptibility Test Methods: Mycobacteria, Nocarida, and Other Actinomycetes. In: Versalovic J, ed. *Manual of Clinical Microbiology*, 10th ed. Washington, DC: ASM, 2011.

CHAPTER 8

MYCOLOGY

Geraldine S. Hall, PhD

This chapter presents information on the more commonly isolated fungal organisms in regard to their usual appearance on direct smears. The table below is not an all-inclusive list but represents the most common fungal organisms likely to be found in human clinical samples. It is divided by the fungal groups of yeasts and molds and further divided by how these appear and would be reported out by clinical laboratories. In addition, the table includes relevant information about each organism's key characteristics with emphasis on how long it should take for cultures to become positive.

The flow diagrams in Figures 8-1 and 8-2 below are to assist in understanding what the clinical laboratory means when they report results of direct smear on clinical samples. These diagrams should help infection preventionists determine what organism(s) is most likely to be seen in the sample on the day it is collected. This in turn should enable clinical personnel to make rapid decisions about treatment options even before the cultures confirm the diagnosis. These results should be used in conjunction with clinical and pathological findings, if available.

The references at the end of the chapter can be used to find additional information on the fungal organisms listed and additional information if an organism is encountered in practice but is not included in this chapter.

Figure 8-1: How to interpret fungal smear results

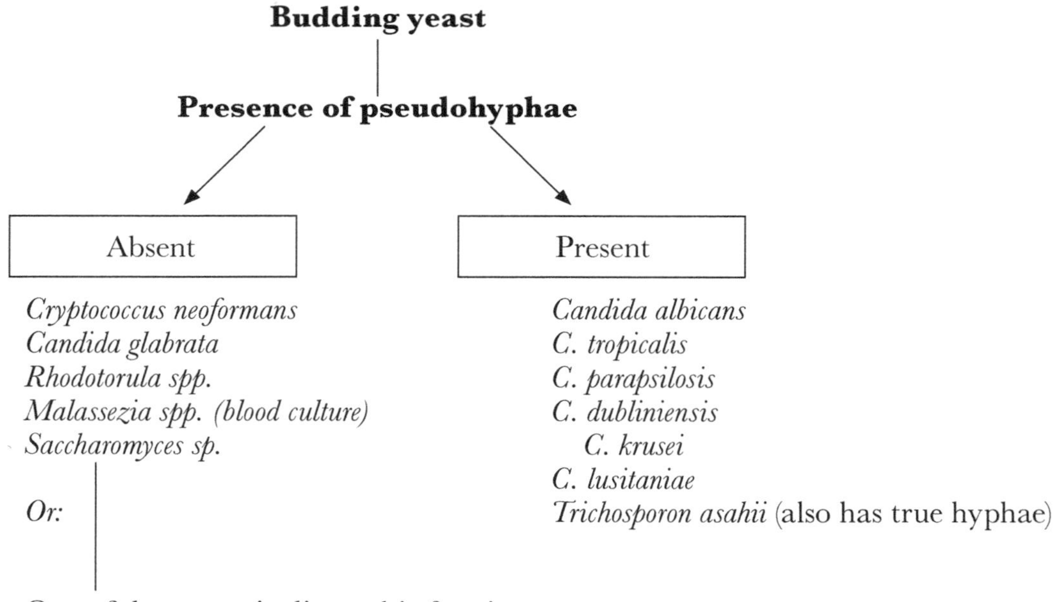

Cryptococcus neoformans
Candida glabrata
Rhodotorula spp.
Malassezia spp. (blood culture)
Saccharomyces sp.

Candida albicans
C. tropicalis
C. parapsilosis
C. dubliniensis
C. krusei
C. lusitaniae
Trichosporon asahii (also has true hyphae)

Or:

One of the systemic dimorphic fungi:
Histoplasma capsulatum (small budding yeast cells in macrophages; in bone marrow, sputum, bronchoalveolar lavage, spleen, liver)
Blastomyces dermatitidis (broad-based budding yeast cells, especially in respiratory or skin specimens)
Coccidioides immitis (spherules found especially in pulmonary specimens or cerebro-spinal fluid)
Paracoccidioides brasiliensis (multiple budding yeast cells)
Sporothrix schenckii (skin specimens in particular with football-shaped budding yeast cells)
Penicillium marneffei (nonbudding, but mimic yeast cells)

Figure 8-2: How to interpret fungal smear results

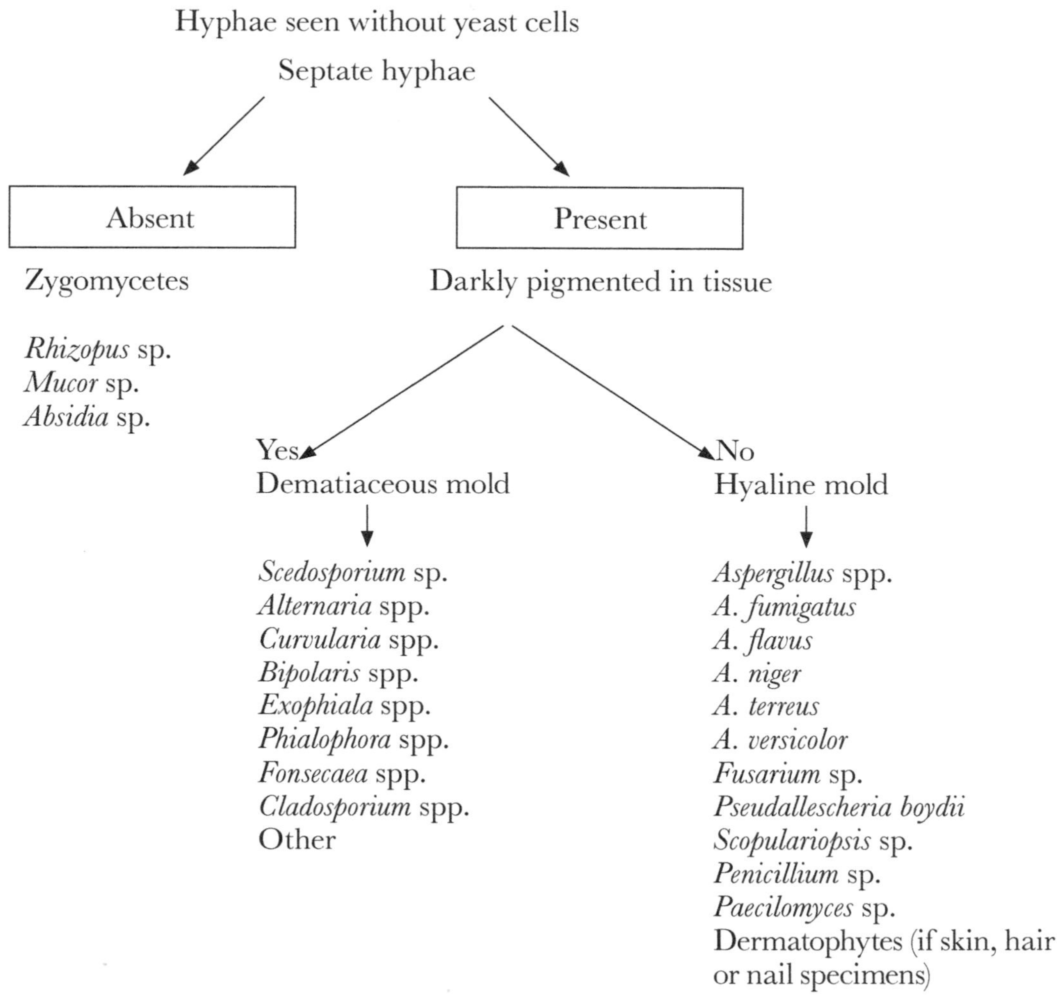

Table 8-1: Overview of Fungal Smears by Organism

Groups of fungi	Species	Epidemiology	Diseases	Test Type	Specimen	Time to results	Appearance in smears	Interpretation	Key points
Candida spp.	*Candida albicans*	• Ubiquitous • Normal gastrointestinal (GI) and skin flora	• Most common in skin and subcutaneous abscesses and wounds • Urinary tract infections • Fungemia and other infections Can cause disseminated disease	Fungal culture and smear	• Blood culture • Swab of mouth, skin • Cerebrospinal fluid (CSF) • Aspirate of abscess or tissue; body fluids; urine • Not usually requested nor looked for in stool	1–2 days	Budding yeast cells and pseudohyphae	• White, usually mucoid-looking colonies; may contain "feet" or evidence of pseudohyphae • Produce chlamydospores terminally on cornmeal agar • Germ-tube positive	
	Candida glabrata	Ubiquitous	Second most common in fungemia and other infections	Fungal culture and smear	• Blood culture • Swab of mouth, skin • CSF • Aspirate of abscess or tissue; urine or other body fluid	1–2 days	• Budding yeast • No pseudohyphae	• White, usually mucoid-looking colonies • Germ-tube negative • No "feet" in culture because it does not produce any pseudohyphae	May be confused in tissue with *H. capsulatum* or *Cryptococcus neoformans*
	Candida tropicalis	Ubiquitous	• Common *Candida* spp. • Often associated with catheter-associated fungemias	Fungal culture and smear	• Blood culture • Swab of mouth, skin • CSF • Aspirate of abscess or tissue; body fluid	1–2 days	Budding yeast cells and pseudohyphae		
	Candida parapsilosis	Ubiquitous	• Common *Candida* spp. • Often associated with catheter-associated fungemias	Fungal culture and smear	• Blood culture • Swab of mouth, skin • CSF • Aspirate of abscess or tissue; body fluid	1–2 days	Budding yeast cells and pseudohyphae		
	Candida dubliniensis	Ubiquitous	May be reported as *C. albicans*	Fungal culture and smear	• Blood culture • Swab of mouth, skin • CSF • Aspirate of abscess or tissue; body fluid	1–2 days	Budding yeast cells and pseudohyphae		

Table 8-1: Overview of Fungal Smears by Organism *(continued)*

Groups of Fungi	Species	Epidemiology	Diseases	Test Type	Specimen	Time to Results	Appearance in Smears	Interpretation	Key Points
Candida spp. *(continued)*	*Candida krusei*	Ubiquitous; perhaps more in hospital environments	Rare, but is a more resistant *Candida* spp., especially to fluconazole	Fungal culture and smear	• Blood culture • Swab of mouth, skin • CSF • Aspirate of abscess or tissue • Body fluid	1–2 days	Budding yeast cells and pseudohyphae		
Cryptococcus sp.	*Cryptococcus neoformans*	• Droppings of birds • Soil	Cause of pneumonia, meningitis, brain abscess, and fungemia	Fungal culture and cryptococcal antigen that can be performed on CSF or serum; serology is available	• Sputum or other respiratory specimens • CSF • Synovial fluid • Blood • Aspirates of skin lesions • Aspirates of tissues • Body fluids	2–3 days	• Budding yeast cell with a prominent capsule around the cell • No pseudohyphae		
	Cryptococcus spp.		• Often a nonpathogen • Can be cause of meningitis or fungemia	Fungal culture and smear		2–3 days	• Budding yeast • No pseudohyphae		
Rhodotorula sp.	*Rhodotorula rubra*	• Soil • Ubiquitous • Hospital environments	Rarely a cause of infections	Fungal culture and smear	• Blood culture • Skin • CSF • Aspirate of abscess or tissue • Body fluid	1–3 days	• Budding yeast • No pseudohyphae	Pink pigmented yeast	
	Other *Rhodotorula* spp.	• Soil • Ubiquitous • Hospital environments	Rarely a cause of infections	Fungal culture and smear	• Blood culture • Skin • CSF • Aspirate of abscess or tissue • Body fluid	1–3 days	• Budding yeast • No pseudohyphae	Nonpigmented	
Saccharomyces sp.	*Saccharomyces cerevisiae*		• Rarely a cause of infections • Common bread and beer yeast	Fungal culture and smear	• Blood culture • Skin • CSF • Aspirate of abscess or tissue • Body fluid	1–2 days	• Budding yeast • No pseudohyphae • May produce ascospores		

Table 8-1: Overview of Fungal Smears by Organism *(continued)*

GROUPS OF FUNGI	SPECIES	EPIDEMIOLOGY	DISEASES	TEST TYPE	SPECIMEN	TIME TO RESULTS	APPEARANCE IN SMEARS	INTERPRETATION	KEY POINTS
Saccharomyces sp. *(continued)*	*Malassezia furfur*	• Worldwide • Normal flora component of skin and sebaceous glands	• Can cause the cutaneous condition known as tinea versicolor • Can also be associated with folliculitis, seborrheic dermatitis, and obstructive dacryocystitis • Can also cause a catheter-associated fungemia in patients receiving total parenteral nutrition with lipid supplementation	Fungal culture and smear	• Blood cultures (labs should be alerted of need to overlay with oil for subcultures of positive bottles) • Skin scrapings	< 1 week	• Budding yeast cells in blood culture smears • May appear as a mixture of budding yeast cells and true hyphae in skin scrapings	• Require oil for growth in the laboratory • Yeast cells are said to resemble "bowling balls"	
Dimorphic molds	*Histoplasma capsulatum*	• Worldwide, but endemic to areas near Mississippi and Ohio River valleys in United States • Endemic in areas of Central and South America, Africa, Australia, India, and Malaysia • Associated with bird (starling) droppings • Can be associated with cleaning out of chicken coops or barns and other farm areas • Spelunking (exploring bat caves) can lead to exposures	Cause of pulmonary disease, fungemia, cutaneous diseases, meningitis, and/or disseminated disease	• Fungal culture and smear • *Histoplasma* antigen in urine • Serology	• Sputum; bronchoalveolar lavage • CSF • Blood • Aspirates of pus from lymph nodes; aspirates from subcutaneous abscesses; tissues; bone marrow; urine or other body fluids	5–15 days but cultures are held up to 4–6 weeks before signing out as negative	• Tissue: small budding yeast cells (3–5 microns) in macrophages or extracellularly • In culture: septate hyphae with small conidia and larger tuberculated macroconidia • Can convert to yeast form at 37°C	• White to tan colonies • Colonies may darken with age	• Pathology will report as small budding yeast cells, consistent with *Histoplasma* • Often seen in macrophages or other cells of the reticulo-endothelial system

Table 8-1: Overview of Fungal Smears by Organism *(continued)*

Groups of fungi	Species	Epidemiology	Diseases	Test type	Specimen	Time to results	Appearance in smears	Interpretation	Key points
Dimorphic molds *(continued)*	*Histoplasma duboisii*	Endemic to the African continent	Cause of cutaneous diseases or bone disease	• Fungal culture and smear • *Histoplasma* antigen in urine • Serology	• Aspirates from subcutaneous abscesses • Synovial fluid or bone	5–15 days but cultures are held up to 4–6 weeks before signing out as negative	• Tissue: small thick-walled budding yeast cells (8–15 microns) in macrophages or extracellularly • In culture: septate hyphae with small conidia and larger tuberculated macroconidia; can convert to yeast form in lab at 37°C	• White to tan colonies • Colonies may darken with age	• Pathology will report as small budding yeast cells, consistent with *Histoplasma* • Often seen in macrophages or other cells of the reticulo-endothelial system
	Blastomyces dermatitidis	• Found worldwide in acidic soil with high nitrogen and organic content • Often cases are seen in individuals near water (Mississippi and Ohio River valleys) or around beaver dams • Endemic to North America, parts of Central and South America • In Canada along the Great Lakes	• Cause of pulmonary disease, fungemia, and/or disseminated disease • Also cutaneous diseases and meningitis	• Fungal culture and smear • Serology • Urinary antigen test being developed	• Sputum • CSF • Abscesses of skin; body fluids • Aspirates of tissues and body fluids; blood	1–2 weeks; cultures will often be held 4–6 weeks before being signed out as negative	• Tissue: larger budding yeast cells with broad-base buds (5–10 microns) and double refractile wall • In culture: septate hyphae with small conidia along the hyphae or connected to it by small conidiophores; can convert to yeast form at 37°C	• White to tan colonies that may darken with age • Colonies may become wrinkled or folded	• The tissue form is often referred to as broad-based buds with a double refractile wall in the pathology report • Although this can be the cause of pulmonary disease like *H. capsulatum*, it is also as likely to be involved as primary cutaneous disease
	Coccidioides immitis	• Found in the soil with a restricted geographical location • Endemic in United States in San Joaquin valley in central and southern California, southern Arizona, New Mexico, and Utah and parts of west Texas • Endemic in northern Mexico and parts of Central and South America	Cause of pulmonary disease, meningitis, bone and joint infections, brain abscesses and disseminated disease	• Fungal culture and smear • Serology	• Sputum; bronchoalveolar lavage • CSF • Synovial fluid • Aspirates of skin lesions, abscesses, tissue; body fluids; blood	< 1 week; often 2–4 days	• Tissue: large spherules (30–50 microns) filled with endospores (2–5 microns) • In culture: septate hyphae broken up into barrel-shaped arthroconidia; cannot convert to yeast form in lab	White, rapid grower filling up agar plate readily	• No yeast form in culture as is seen with other systemic dimorphic fungi • The spherules in tissue are very large, but the endospores can resemble a *H. capsulatum* yeast cell, but without any budding

Table 8-1: Overview of Fungal Smears by Organism (continued)

Groups of Fungi	Species	Epidemiology	Diseases	Test Type	Specimen	Time to Results	Appearance in Smears	Interpretation	Key Points
Dimorphic molds (continued)	Paracoc-cidioides brasiliensis	• Probably the reservoir is soil • Endemic to Central and South America, although most cases come from the latter, especially Brazil, Venezuela, and Colombia • Most common locality is in subtropical upland rain forests	• Cause of pulmonary disease, fungemia, and/or disseminated disease • Also cutaneous diseases and meningitis	Fungal culture and smear	• Sputum • Bronchoalveolar lavage (BAL) • Aspirates of skin lesions, abscesses, tissue; body fluids; blood		• Tissue: large budding yeast with multiple buds • In culture: septate hyphae with small conidia along the hyphae, resembling *B. dermatitidis* • Can convert to yeast form at 37°C	Cream or white dry colonies that become darker with age and more wrinkled and folded	• Resembles *B. dermatitidis* in culture • Cross reacts with probes for *B. dermatitidis* • Pathology report will often refer to appearance of the "mariner's wheel" to describe the yeast forms
	Penicillium marneffei	• Reservoir appears to be decaying organic material and soil • Endemic to northern Thailand (most cases from here) and other Southeast Asian countries • An AIDS-defining illness	Cause of pulmonary disease and/or disseminated disease most often in HIV patients	Culture and smear	• Sputum • BAL, blood • Aspirates, tissues, body fluids	< 1 week; often 2–4 days	• Tissue: ovoid single cells without budding; a "cross-wall or bar" often seen inside of the cell • In culture: septate hyphae with conidiophores and fruiting heads characteristic of all other *Penicillium* spp. • Can convert to yeast-like form at 37°C	Produces a diffusible red pigment on agar plates	• In culture, may resemble any saprophytic *Penicillium* spp., except for production of red pigment • Other species of *Penicillium* may produce a red pigment • Without appropriate travel history or patients coming from endemic areas, unlikely to see this organism in the United States in someone who has never traveled to Southeast Asia

Table 8-1: Overview of Fungal Smears by Organism *(continued)*

Groups of fungi	Species	Epidemiology	Diseases	Test type	Specimen	Time to results	Appearance in smears	Interpretation	Key points
Dimorphic molds *(continued)*	*Sporothrix schenckii*	• Reservoir is soil, organic material • Vegetables and plants • Widespread, but more common in temperate and tropical climates	• Cause of cutaneous and subcutaneous lesions/abscesses after trauma or implantation from organic material like thorns of rose bushes • Rarely pulmonary or disseminated disease (usually only in severely immuno-compromised patients; i.e., AIDS patients)	Fungal culture and smear	• Aspirates of skin or subcutaneous lesions • Skin biopsy; lymph nodes; rarely respiratory or blood specimens	< 1 week; often growth in 2–3 days	• Tissue: oval to "cigar or football-shaped" budding yeast cells • In culture: septate hyphae with conidia found as a "collarette" along the hyphae on short projections or at end of long projection (conidiophore) resembling a flower; can convert this mold form to a yeast form at 37°C	• The mold form is often very dark brown-black • Referred to as a dematiaceous mold	Tissues are rarely positive for the yeast form, a term referred to as "pauci-" or low yield
Zygomycetes (Mucorm-ycosis)	*Rhizopus oryzae* and other spp.		• Cutaneous and subcutaneous infections • Pulmonary disease • Disseminated disease in immuno-compromised hosts • Brain abscesses • Endophthalmitis (diabetics)	• Fungal culture and smear • May want to alert lab of possibility because specimen processing should be done by mincing rather than grinding to maintain the integrity of the mold	• Aspirates of cutaneous lesions; respiratory specimens including sputum and BAL • Body fluids and tissues • Rarely blood cultures	1–2 days	• Smear: aseptate hyphae • Culture: white fluffy "lid-lifter"	• Very rapid growth • Called one of the lid-lifters because, if not taped down, plates can be lifted by the mycelium • Has been associated with contaminated adhesive bandages and other fomites	• Characteristic in culture: presence of aseptate hyphae • Rhizoids present at end of sporangiophore
	Rhizopus niger		• Cutaneous and subcutaneous infections • Pulmonary disease • Disseminated disease in immuno-compromised hosts • Brain abscesses • Endophthalmitis (diabetics)	• Fungal culture and smear • May want to alert lab of possibility because specimen processing should be done by mincing rather than grinding to maintain the integrity of the mold	• Aspirates of cutaneous lesions • Respiratory specimens including sputum and BAL • Body fluids and tissues • Rarely blood cultures	1–2 days	• Smear: aseptate hyphae • Culture: white fluffy with black "spots" (spores), "lid-lifter"	• Very rapid growth • Called one of the lid-lifters because, if not taped down, plates can be lifted by the mycelium • Has been associated with contaminated adhesive bandages and other fomites	• Characteristic in culture: presence of aseptate hyphae • Rhizoids present at end of sporangiophore • Black spores

Table 8-1: Overview of Fungal Smears by Organism (*continued*)

Groups of fungi	Species	Epidemiology	Diseases	Test Type	Specimen	Time to results	Appearance in smears	Interpretation	Key Points
Zygomycetes (Mucormycosis) (*continued*)	*Mucor* spp.		• Cutaneous and subcutaneous infections • Pulmonary disease • Disseminated disease in immuno-compromised hosts • Brain abscesses • Endophthalmitis (diabetics)	• Fungal culture and smear • May want to alert lab of possibility because specimen processing should be done by mincing rather than grinding to maintain the integrity of the mold	• Aspirates of cutaneous lesions; respiratory specimens including sputum and BAL • Body fluids and tissues • Rarely blood cultures	1–2 days	• Smear: aseptate hyphae • Culture: white fluffy "lid-lifter"	• Very rapid growth • Called one of the lid-lifters because, if not taped down, plates can be lifted by the mycelium • Has been associated with contaminated adhesive bandages and other fomites	• Characteristic in culture: presence of aseptate hyphae • No rhizoids present
	Absidia sp.		• Cutaneous and subcutaneous infections • Pulmonary disease • Disseminated disease in immuno-compromised hosts • Brain abscesses • Endophthalmitis (diabetics)	• Fungal culture and smear • May want to alert lab of possibility because specimen processing should be done by mincing rather than grinding to maintain the integrity of the mold	• Aspirates of cutaneous lesions; respiratory specimens including sputum and BAL • Body fluids and tissues • Rarely blood cultures	1–2 days	• Smear: aseptate hyphae • Culture: white fluffy "lid-lifter"	• Very rapid growth • Called one of the lid-lifters because, if not taped down, plates can be lifted by the mycelium • Has been associated with contaminated adhesive bandages and other fomites	• Characteristic in culture: presence of aseptate hyphae • Rhizoids present internodally (i.e., between sporangiophores)
Hyaline molds	*Aspergillus fumigatus*	• Ubiquitous in environment • Airborne mold • Found in compost piles, soil, including in potted plants	• Primary pulmonary disease • Disseminated disease • Can infect any organ, especially in hematology-oncology and transplant patients	Fungal culture and smear	• Respiratory specimens including sputum and BAL • Blood cultures (rarely positive) • Tissues and body fluids • A galactomannan serum antigen test might be ordered to aid in the diagnosis of disseminated infections with *A. fumigatus*	1–2 days	• Smear: septate hyphae at 45 angles • Culture: flat mycelium with blue-green color • Reverse = white	• Rapid growth • Of hyaline mold with characteristic fruiting heads in which conidia cover three-fourths of the top of the conidial head	Most common of the pathogenic hyaline molds

Table 8-1: Overview of Fungal Smears by Organism (*continued*)

Groups of Fungi	Species	Epidemiology	Diseases	Test Type	Specimen	Time to Results	Appearance in Smears	Interpretation	Key Points
Hyaline molds (*continued*)	*Aspergillus flavus*	• Ubiquitous in environment • Airborne mold • Found in compost piles, soil, including in potted plants	• Primary pulmonary disease • Disseminated disease • Can infect any organ, especially in hematology-oncology and transplant patients	Fungal culture and smear	• Respiratory specimens including sputum and BAL • Blood cultures (rarely positive) • Tissues and body fluids	1–2 days	• Smear: septate hyphae at 45 angles • Culture: flat mycelium with yellow-green color • Reverse = white	Rapid growth or hyaline mold with characteristic fruiting head	Second most common of pathogenic *Aspergillus* spp.
	Aspergillus niger	Ubiquitous in environment	• Otitis externa • Can cause pulmonary disease or colonization	Fungal culture and smear	• Swab of external ear • Sputum and BAL • Tissues and body fluids	1–2 days	• Smear: septate hyphae at 45 angles • Culture: flat mycelium with black conidia produced and hence appearance of culture is "black and white" with a reverse of white	• Rapid growth of white mold that has characteristic black conidia throughout the top surface appearing as black granules • Characteristic fruiting head	Common lab contaminant as well as potentially significant *Aspergillus* sp.
	Aspergillus terreus	Ubiquitous in environment	Pulmonary disease, but can be associated with other body sites as colonizer or pathogen	Fungal culture and smear	• Respiratory specimens including sputum and BAL • Blood cultures (rarely positive) • Tissues and body fluids	1–2 days	• Smear: septate hyphae at 45 angles • Culture: flat mycelium with cinnamon-brown colony color, with a reverse of white	Rapid growth	• Rarely isolated from human specimens, but can be a pathogen • It is reportedly increasing in incidence • This species of *Aspergillus* is often resistant to common antifungal agents, like amphotericin
	Aspergillus versicolor	Ubiquitous in environment	Pulmonary disease, but can be associated with other body sites as colonizer or pathogen	Fungal culture and smear	• Respiratory specimens including sputum and BAL • Blood cultures (rarely positive) • Tissues and body fluids	> 2 days	• Smear: septate hyphae at 45 angles • Culture: flat mycelium with greenish-tan or other nonblack colony color, with a reverse of white	Slower growth than other *Aspergillus* spp.	Rarely isolated from human specimens, but can be a pathogen

Table 8-1: Overview of Fungal Smears by Organism *(continued)*

Groups of Fungi	Species	Epidemiology	Diseases	Test Type	Specimen	Time to Results	Appearance in Smears	Interpretation	Key Points
Hyaline molds *(continued)*	*Fusarium* spp.	• Ubiquitous in environment • Found in soil • Can be a plant pathogen • Can produce toxins in plants and in humans	• Pulmonary disease, fungemia, and/or disseminated disease in the immuno-compromised, often neutropenic, patient • Can also cause keratitis, localized organ or tissue infections; may be responsible for nail infections as well	Fungal culture and smear	• Respiratory including sputum and BAL • Blood and other sterile body fluids • Tissues • Corneal scrapings (often associated with contact lens users)	Fast growing; < 1 week usually	• Smear: septate hyphae at 45 angles • Culture: colonies start out white and can become a variety of colors including creamy white to pink, blue, reddish, purple or blue-green; texture of colony can be "felt-like" or cottony	Rapid growth of hyaline mold with "canoe-shaped macroconidia"	• *Fusarium* is usually second in incidence of isola-tion to *Aspergillus* spp. from clinical samples as a pathogen • *Fusarium* can also look very much like *Aspergillus* spp. in tissue smears • *Fusarium*, if the pathogen of dis-seminated disease, is also more likely to be isolated from blood cultures than is *Aspergillus* spp.

Table 8-1: Overview of Fungal Smears by Organism *(continued)*

Groups of fungi	Species	Epidemiology	Diseases	Test Type	Specimen	Time to results	Appearance in smears	Interpretation	Key points
Hyaline molds *(continued)*	*Pseudoallescheria boydii (Scedosporium apiospermum)*	Ubiquitous in environment in soil, stagnant and polluted water, sewage, plants, and decaying vegetation	• Pulmonary disease, fungemia, and/or disseminated disease in the immuno-compromised patient • Can also cause localized organ or tissue infections	Fungal culture and smear	• Respiratory including sputum and BAL • Blood and other sterile body fluids • Tissues • Fluid or tissue from cases of mycetoma	Usually grows out in 3–5 days	• Smear: septate hyphae at 45 angles • Culture: colonies start out white and becomes a mousey-gray color on surface and white on reverse of culture plate	Growth of gray colonies with characteristic septate hyphae and oval conidia on short stalks	• *P. boydii,* (or its asexual name, *Scedosporium apiospermum*) can be clinically significant when isolated from pulmonary specimens of patient with high risk: leukemia and lymphoma patients, patients with chronic obstructive pulmonary disease, systemic lupus erythematosus, patients receiving immuno-suppressants, HIV patients • Can also cause disseminated disease in immuno-compromised patients • The most common cause of eumycetoma in the United States

Table 8-1: Overview of Fungal Smears by Organism (continued)

GROUPS OF FUNGI	SPECIES	EPIDEMIOLOGY	DISEASES	TEST TYPE	SPECIMEN	TIME TO RESULTS	APPEARANCE IN SMEARS	INTERPRETATION	KEY POINTS
Hyaline molds (continued)	*Paecilomyces* spp., most commonly *P. variotii* and *P. lilacinus*	Found worldwide as soil saprophytes, insect parasites	Rare cases of pulmonary disease, keratitis, or endocarditis, cutaneous and subcutaneous infections, cellulitis, sinusitis	Fungal culture and smear	Could be isolated from any specimen a saprophyte or pathogen: keratitis, cutaneous, and subcutaneous infections, pulmonary infections, sinusitis, cellulitis, endocarditis, and fungemia	1–2 days (*P. variotii*); slower growth (≥ 1 week) for *P. lilacinus*, for example	• Rarely seen directly in tissue or smears; however, would resemble *Aspergillus* spp., although would probably not be found invading blood vessels • Cultures: colonies start out with and may become brightly pigmented, nonblack or brown; reverse of plate remains nonpigmented	Growth of white colonies that can become lightly pigments such as yellowish-brown to orange (*P. variotii*) to violet (*P. lilacinus*)	• There are > 40 species; the most common are *P. lilacinus* and *P. variotii* • Can be often isolated in clinical laboratories as contaminants or can be found in patient specimens as a result of colonization • Can be seen in smears, grow in sufficient numbers to be a pathogen
	Scopulariopsis spp., most commonly *S. brevicaulis* and *S. brumptii*	Common soil fungi and agents of deterioration	• Rare cases of pulmonary disease, keratitis or endocarditis, cutaneous and subcutaneous infections, cellulitis, sinusitis • They are the most common mold responsible for nondermatophyte nail infections	Fungal culture and smear	Most commonly specimens would be nails (tinea pedis), pulmonary specimens including sputum and BAL or lung tissue	3–5 days	• Rarely seen directly in tissue or smears; however, would resemble *Aspergillus* spp., although would probably not be found invading blood vessels. • Cultures: colonies start out as white and can become gray; some species may produce dark brown to black colonies	Colonies are white and have characteristic fruiting structures, called annelides from which the conidia are produced	There are many species, but few have been found in clinical specimens

Table 8-1: Overview of Fungal Smears by Organism *(continued)*

Groups of Fungi	Species	Epidemiology	Diseases	Test Type	Specimen	Time to Results	Appearance in Smears	Interpretation	Key Points
Hyaline molds *(continued)*	*Penicillium* spp.	• Ubiquitous in soil and decaying plant matter • Very common laboratory contaminants	Very rare cases of pulmonary disease	Culture and smear	• Can be isolated from any specimens, although most commonly in BAL or sputum and nail specimens • Usually they are there as contaminant or colonizer of patient; rarely implicated in disease	1–3 days	• Rarely seen directly in tissue or smears • Would resemble *Aspergillus* spp., although would probably not be found invading blood vessels • Cultures: colonies start out as white and often become green to blue-green colonies; reverse is not black	Colonies are white and have characteristic fruiting structures that are often referred to as "fingers"	There are many species
	Dermato-phytes	• Some are found in soil (geophilic strains) • Some in animals (zoophilic strains) or anthropophilic (found in humans only)	Tinea infections of hair, skin, and nails	Fungal culture and smear	• Hair, skin, nails • Rarely seen in pulmonary specimens	1–4 weeks	Smear: septate hyphae broken up into arthroconidia	• Colonies are white and may develop light-colored pigments with time • Reverse may be yellow, tan, or red, but never black or brown	There are three main genera: *Microsporum*, *Trichophyton*, and *Epidermophyton*
Dematiaceous (darkly pigmented) molds		• Found in the soil and on decaying plant materials • Geographically may be seen more in warm than temperate or colder climates	• Chromo-blastomycosis, a cutaneous disease often seen in tropical and subtropical climates • Rarely may be involved in pulmonary disease • Sinusitis • Very rarely disseminated disease in immuno-compromised hosts	Fungal culture and smear	• Cutaneous and subcutaneous tissue, lesion material • Rarely in pulmonary specimens	1–4 weeks	• Smear: septate hyphae with presence of melanin (brown deposits) • May be positive for specific melanin stains	Colonies may begin as white and tiny, but with age develop a black-to-brown color on top surface and reverse side of petri dish	• There are many genera and species • Some such as *Alternaria* and *Curvularia* are rarely involved in clinical disease, but rather appear as lab contaminants • Others like *Fonsecaea*, *Exophiala*, *Phialophora*, or *Cladosporium* can be pathogens from traumatic implantation or as opportunists in the immuno-compromised host

References

Fothergill AW. Medically Significant Fungi. In: Mahon CR, Lehman DC, Manuselis G, eds. *Textbook of Diagnostic Microbiology*, 4th ed. Maryland Heights: WB Saunders Company, 2011: 603-638.

Larone DH. *Medically Important Fungi: A Guide to Identification*, 4th ed. Washington, DC: ASM Press, 2002.

Miller JM. *A Guide to Specimen Management in Clinical Microbiology*, 2nd ed. Washington, DC: ASM Press, 1999.

Mycoses study group. Doctor Fungus Website. 2007. Available at: http://www.doctorfungus.org/mycoses/MSG/msg_index.php. Accessed December 18, 2011.

Versalovic J, Carroll KC, Funke G, Jorgensen JH, Landry ML, Warnock DW, eds. *Manual of Clinical Microbiology*, 10th ed. Washington, DC: ASM Press, 2011.

Winn W, Allen S, Janda W, Koneman E, Procop G, Schreckenberger P, et al., eds. *Koneman's Color Atlas and Textbook of Clinical Microbiology*, 6th ed. Philadelphia: Lippincott Williams & Wilkins, 2006.

Chapter 9

Parasitology

Jeanne Dickman, MT(ASCP), CIC

This chapter describes the field of parasitology as it applies to infection prevention. A parasite is an organism that lives in or on another (the host) from which it obtains nourishment. The host does not benefit from the association and is often harmed by it.

Most parasitic infections are spread by the fecal-oral route or by arthropods (mosquitoes, etc.). The exception to this would be those transmitted by direct contact, such as lice and scabies, which have been identified in healthcare outbreaks. In general, parasitic infections are not commonly healthcare-associated but can be a significant problem in extended or residential care facilities for patients with physical or mental disabilities. Due to the nature of these patient populations, challenges with crowding, environmental sanitation, and personal hygiene can lead to rapid dissemination and endemic occurrence of a large variety of parasitic infections. For more information about specific parasites, including mode of transmission and infections caused by them, please refer to APIC's *Ready Reference for Microbes*.

The following tables are arranged by laboratory tests describing the parasites. The tables are designed to enhance the knowledge of the infection preventionist (IP) as he/she reviews laboratory results for their patient populations. The tables describe what tests are useful, when they should be performed, and what the results might mean. The IP is encouraged to discuss further questions with their microbiology laboratorians when issues arise.

Table 9-1: Overview of Parasitology Tests

General Category	Laboratory Test	Indications	Specific Microbes	Specimen	Frequency	Interpretation	Advantages/Disadvantages	Key Points
Microscopic	Ova and parasite (O&P) direct wet mount	Diarrhea	Protozoan trophozoites and cysts, helminth eggs, and larvae	• Stool in clean, dry, tightly sealed container or collection kit • Specimens containing barium are unacceptable • Must wait 7–10 days after barium administration	Three specimens, a day or two apart within 10 days of each other	Detection of diagnostic stage of parasite		
	O&P, concentrated	Diarrhea	Protozoan cysts, helminth eggs, and larvae	Stool, same limitations as above	Three specimens, a day or two apart within 10 days	Detection of diagnostic stage of parasite	Protozoan trophozoites will not survive concentration	
	O&P, permanently stained smears	Diarrhea	Protozoan trophozoites and cysts, helminth eggs, and larvae	Stool, same limitations as above	Three specimens, a day or two apart within 10 days	Detection of diagnostic stage of parasite		
	Modified Kinyoun acid fast stain	Diarrhea	*Cryptosporidium, Isopspora belii, Cyclospora cayetanansis*	Stool, same limitations as above	Three specimens, a day or two apart within 10 days	Detection of oocysts		
	Cellophane tape prep/collection kits	Perineal itching	*Enterobius vermicularis* (pinworms)	Tape prep of perineal area	Collect first thing in the morning before use of bathroom	Detection of ova	Three to five consecutive negative preps to rule out infection	• Common intestinal helminthic infection • Symptoms include perianal itching, disturbed sleep, irritability • Eggs in an indoor environment remain infective for two weeks
	Microscopic exam	Diarrhea	*Giardia, Strongyloides, Fasciola hepatica* or *Clonorchis sinensis* ova, *Cryptosporidium* or *Isospora* oocysts	Duodenal aspirates or duodenal capsule (Entero-Test)	Consult laboratory	Detection of diagnostic stage of parasite	Useful when clinical symptoms are suggestive of infection and routine O&P is negative	
	Microscopic exam	Diarrhea	Amebiasis, *Cryptosporidium*	Sigmoidoscopy aspirate or scraping	Done only after at least three negative O&P	Detection of diagnostic stage of parasite	• Examination of fresh specimen by trained microscopist to differentiate nonpathogenic amoebae and macrophages • Reference lab services may be requird	Presence of trophozoites containing red blood cells indicative of invasive amoebiasis

Table 9-1: Overview of Parasitology Tests (*continued*)

General Category	Laboratory Test	Indications	Specific Microbes	Specimen	Frequency	Interpretation	Advantages/Disadvantages	Key Points
	Microscopic exam	Hematuria	*Schistosoma haematobium* ova, *Enterobius vermicularis* ova, *Trichomonas vaginalis* trophozoites	Urine	Early morning specimen	Detection of diagnostic stage of parasite	Urine filtration useful for *S. haematobium* infections	
	Microscopic exam	Vaginal/urethral discharge	*Trichomonas vaginalis* trophozoites	Vaginal and urethral discharge	Consult laboratory	Detection of trophozoites	• Organisms can be seen on a Papanicolaou smear • Polymerase chain reaction (PCR) test available but insufficiently reliable for routine use	
	Microscopic exam	Cough/bloody sputum	Migrating larval stages of hookworm, *Ascaris* and *Strongyloides stercoralis*, *Paragonimus westermani* ova	Sputum	Consult laboratory	Detection of diagnostic stage of parasite		• Asacria pulmonary manifestations caused by larval migration (mainly during reinfestation) • Characterized by wheezing, coughing, fever, eosinophilia, pulmonary infiltration
	Microscopic exam	Fever of unknown origin/ temperature spikes, malaria	*Plasmodium*, *Babesia*, *Trypanosoma*, some microfilarea	Blood from fingerstick or ethylenediaminetetraacetic acid (EDTA) blood draw, thick and thin smears	Consult laboratory	Detection of parasite in blood smear	Best results when processed within 1 hour	If patient has traveled to malaria endemic area, dates and area traveled are important to diagnosis
	Microscopic exam	Diarrhea, abdominal pain	*Entamoeba histolytica*	Liver biopsy	Consult laboratory		• IgM serological tests, particularly immunodiffusion and **enzyme-linked immunosorbent assay (ELISA)**, are very useful in the diagnosis of invasive disease • Ultrasound and computed tomography scans beneficial in locating amoebic liver abscesses	• Dissemination via the bloodstream may occur and produce abscesses of the liver, less commonly the lung or brain • The presence of trophozoites containing red blood cells is indicative of invasive amoebiasis
	Microscopic exam	Skin sores	*Leishmania* spp.	Tissue biopsy	Consult laboratory			

Table 9-1: Overview of Parasitology Tests *(continued)*

General Category	Laboratory Test	Indications	Specific Microbes	Specimen	Frequency	Interpretation	Advantages/Disadvantages	Key Points
Immunology	Serology, Enzyme immmunoassay, Immunofluorescence antibody	Generally asymptomatic or mild flu-like symptoms	*Toxoplasma*	Blood	Consult laboratory	Detection of IgM, IgG antibodies	Useful in diagnosis of invasive disease	
	Serology, Enzyme immmunoassay, Immunofluorescence antibody	Generally asymptomatic; in some cases, muscle soreness, fever, edema of upper eyelids	*Trichinella*	Blood	Consult laboratory	Detection of IgM, IgG antibodies	Useful in diagnosis of invasive disease	
	Serology, Enzyme immmunoassay, Immunofluorescence antibody	Diarrhea	*Amebiasis*	Blood	Consult laboratory	Detection of IgM, IgG antibodies	Useful in diagnosis of extraintestinal amoebiasis, liver abscess, and invasive disease	
	Enzyme immunoassay, direct fluorescent antibody	Diarrhea	*Giardia, Cryptosporidium,* Amebiasis	Stool	Consult laboratory	Detection of antigen		Problems with sensitivity and specificity
	Enzyme immunoassay, direct fluorescent antibody	Vaginal/urethral discharge	*Trichomonas*	Vaginal/urethral discharge	Consult laboratory	Detection of antigen		Problems with sensitivity and specificity
	Enzyme immunoassay	Fever of unknown origin; for Wuchereria, painful lymph nodes	*Plasmodium, Wuchereria*	Blood	Consult laboratory	Detection of antigen	Used where malaria endemic	
Ectoparasites	Exam	Skin infection, pediculosis	*Pediculus humanus* (head lice)	Insect		Detection of insect		Common parasites to infect humans
	Microscopic exam	Skin infection, pediculosis	*Pediculus humanus corporis* (body lice)	Insect		Detection of insect		Common parasites to infect humans
	Microscopic exam	Skin infection, pediculosis	*Phthirus pubis* (crab lice)	Insect		Detection of insect		Common parasites to infect humans
	Microscopic exam	Skin infection	*Sarcoptes scabiei* (scabies)	Skin scrapings		Detection of mites, eggs, and fecal pellets		Common parasites to infect humans

References

Forbes BA, Sahm DF, Weissfeld AS. *Bailey and Scott's Diagnostic Microbiology,* 12th ed. St. Louis: Mosby, 2007.

Heymann DL. *Control of Communicable Diseases Manual,* 19th ed. Washington, DC: American Public Health Association, 2008.

Mahon CR, Lehman DC, Manuselis G. *Textbook of Diagnostic Microbiology,* 4th ed. Maryland Heights: Saunders/Elsevier, 2011.

Additional Resources

Brooks K. *Ready Reference for Microbes,* 3rd ed. Washington, DC: Association for Professionals in Infection Control and Epidemiology, 2012.

Chapter 10

Virology

Lynn Fine, PhD, MPH, CIC

Human viral infections affect all ages and include a wide range of severity. They may be acute or chronic, be recurrent, or elicit lifelong immunity. They are acquired through various routes via contact with other humans, animals, or the environment; they present as various syndromes and have to be rapidly distinguished from bacterial and other infectious and noninfectious etiologies to facilitate appropriate clinical management.

The emphasis and priorities of diagnostic virology laboratories is constantly changing in response to the availability of rapid diagnostic methods, the identification of new viruses many of which are non- or poorly culturable, the increasing availability of effective antiviral agents, the emergence of antiviral resistance, the increasing number of immunocompromised patients in whom opportunistic viral infections are life-threatening, and the cost-effectiveness of performing diagnostic testing.

Routine viral diagnostics include techniques for indirect and direct detection of viruses. Indirect detection is performed by serological studies. Techniques for direct detection of viruses include detection of viral antigens, molecular components, or by isolation of the organism in culture. Moreover, it must be taken into consideration that reliable viral diagnostics depends on preanalytic issues such as the choice of correct specimen, optimal sampling time with regard to the course of the disease, and both time and conditions of specimen transport to the laboratory.

This section reviews testing methodologies for common and uncommon viral pathogens, specimen requirements, and the advantages and disadvantages of each. Also included are result interpretations and testing frequency suggestions. It is the hope that this will serve as a reference to the infection preventionist who, on any given day, has to interpret test outcomes and make recommendations regarding patient placement and exposures based on these results.

Table 10-1: Overview of Testing Methodologies for Viral Pathogens

Test type	Indications	Specific microbes	Specimen	Frequency	Interpretation	Advantages/ disadvantages	Key points
Viral culture	• Viral culture offers the broadest approach to identifying a viral agent • Cultures should be obtained as early as possible after onset of illness	Adenovirus, cytomegalovirus (CMV), enterovirus, herpes simplex virus (HSV), influenza A and B, parainfluenza, respiratory syncytial virus (RSV), rhinovirus, rotavirus, varicella zoster virus (VZV), severe acute respiratory syndrome coronavirus (SARS-CoV), coxsackievirus, echoviruses, herpes group viruses, measles, mumps, and polio	• Specimen swab must be placed in viral transport media • Dacron-tipped, rayon-tipped, or flocked swabs with plastic or aluminum shafts are acceptable • Calcium alginate swabs are inhibitory to HSV and should NOT be used for viral culture collection • Wooden-shafted swabs are not recommended because wooden swabs can contain toxins and formaldehydes that inhibit virus and chlamydia recovery; wooden swabs also absorb transport media, thereby reducing the amount of fluid for inoculation onto cell cultures • Appropriate specimens for culture vary according to syndrome and suspected agents	Acute phase of illness	Positive/negative • Varies with virus, specimen source, and clinical setting; interpretation of positive viral culture results • Latent viruses can reactivate with or without symptoms (e.g., CMV, HSV, VZV, and adenovirus) • Isolation of most viruses occurs only with acute infection when virus excretion is highest	• Considered gold standard in most cases • Long turnaround time • Not all viruses can be cultured • Useful when diagnosis is uncertain • Viral cultures can be performed alone or combined with several antigen detection assays to yield a rapid preliminary result	• Turnaround time will depend on site being cultured • Not all virology laboratories have the capability to grow all viruses • Not all viruses can be cultured
Molecular amplification (hybrid capture)	Diagnosis of high-risk human papilloma virus (HPV) types associated with increased risk of cervical cancer	HPV	Cervical or vaginal specimens (not U.S. Food and Drug Administration–approved for male specimens)	After initial diagnosis made by abnormal Papanicolaou smear	Positive/negative • Can be semiquantitative	Detects the following high-risk types of HPV: 16, 18, 31, 33, 35, 39, 45, 51, 52, 56, 58, 59, and 68; ages 30 and older	Useful in unvaccinated female patients

Table 10-1: Overview of Testing Methodologies for Viral Pathogens *(continued)*

Test type	Indications	Specific microbes	Specimen	Frequency	Interpretation	Advantages/ disadvantages	Key points
Molecular amplification (polymerase chain reaction [PCR])	Diagnosis of encephalitis due to infectious etiologies	Adenovirus, West Nile virus, systemic lupus erythematosis, extracellular enveloped *virus*, Cache Valley and California serogroup viruses, enterovirus, HSV 1 and 2, VZV, Epstein-Barr virus (EBV), human herpesvirus 6 (HHV-6), CMV, John Cunningham virus (JC virus)	Cerebrospinal fluid	Acute phase of illness	Positive/negative	• Methodology should be used for diagnosing central nervous system infections • HSV DNA can be detected immediately after the onset of neurological symptoms, after the initiation of acyclovir therapy, and up to 3 weeks after the onset of symptoms	Enterovirus season July to October
Molecular amplification (PCR)	Amplification of viral genetic material	Adenovirus, BK virus, HHV-6, HHV-8, HSV, JC virus, parvovirus, VZV, metapneumovirus, SARS-CoV, vaccinia, norovirus	Plasma, serum, tissue, nasal wash, urine	Acute phase of illness	Positive/negative	• Can be used for viral genotyping/ resistance monitoring (CMV, human immunodeficiency virus [HIV], hepatitis C virus [HCV]) • Virus isolation is site-specific • Extremely sensitive/ specific	
Molecular amplification (quantitative PCR)	Quantification of viral load	CMV, EBV, hepatitis B virus, HCV, HIV, BK virus	Plasma or serum (unacceptable for HIV testing)	Initial diagnosis and throughout treatment	• Ranges for viral loads will be virus-specific • Reported copies/mL	• Can be used to monitor initiation or effectiveness of therapy and disease progression • Not recommended for diagnosing HIV infection	
Fluorescent antibody	Nonculture detection of viral infection	VZV, HSV 1 and 2, CMV	• Vesicle fluid for VZV • Antigenemia assay performed on blood for CMV • Can confirm HSV subtypes 1 and 4 • Can also be performed on respiratory specimens	Acute phase of illness	Positive/negative	• Rapid turnaround time • Can detect nonviable virus allowing for rapid identification and can identify infection/ colonization of unculturable organisms	

Table 10-1: Overview of Testing Methodologies for Viral Pathogens *(continued)*

Test type	Indications	Specific microbes	Specimen	Frequency	Interpretation	Advantages/ disadvantages	Key points
Enzyme immunoassay (EIA)	• Can be used for detection of antigens in stool • Rapid screening tool for some viruses	RSV, influenza A and B, rotavirus, adenovirus	Nasopharyngeal and other respiratory specimens, stool, serum	Acute phase of illness	Positive/negative	• Rapid turnaround time • Can detect nonviable virus • Influenza and RSV EIAs are good screening tests but negative tests should be followed up with culture or PCR • Positive HIV EIAs must be confirmed by Western blot	For influenza, not H/N-specific

References

Kudesia G, Wreghitt TG. *Clinical and Diagnostic Virology*. Cambridge: Cambridge University Press, 2009.

Persing DH. *Molecular Microbiology: Diagnostic Principles and Practice*, 2nd ed. Washington, DC: ASM Press, 2011.

Richman DD, Whitley RJ, Hayden FG. *Clinical Virology*. Washington, DC: ASM Press, 2009.

Stephenson JR, Warnes A. *Diagnostic Virology Protocols*. Totowa: Humana Press, 2010.

Chapter 11

Other Microbiology Contributions

Justin Smyer, MT(ASCP), MPH

Additional Contributors:
Jill Midgett, MT, SM(ASCP)

Now more than ever, the microbiology laboratory is the first line of detection in the event of new emerging pathogens and antimicrobial resistance. With the increasing availability of sophisticated technologies to rapidly diagnose and treat infections, the roles of clinical microbiology laboratories in infection prevention are dynamically changing beyond the traditional methods of testing. In an era with enhanced focus on healthcare-associated infections (HAIs), infection preventionists are increasingly relying on the microbiology laboratory for a number of services beyond regular culture and sensitivity testing including development of antibiograms, environmental testing, health department reporting, and support in surveillance and outbreak investigations.

Antimicrobial susceptibility testing (AST) is highly complex testing, as categorized by the Clinical Laboratory Improvement Amendments (CLIA). The performance standards and interpretive guidelines for AST are defined by the Clinical and Laboratory Standards Institute (CLSI) through an evidence-based consensus process. Additionally, in 2002, CLSI published the first guidance document (M39-A) for standardizing the statistical analysis of cumulative AST data called an antibiogram. Clinical microbiology laboratories accredited by the College of American Pathologists (CAP) are required to create and distribute an antibiogram annually. Antibiograms can provide information needed to establish antibiotic usage recommendations, rules, and restrictions (e.g., in the case of healthcare-associated *Clostridium difficile*). They can also be useful in deciding where to focus educational efforts as they can be broken down from a hospital-wide to a unit-specific perspective. See Chapter 11 for additional information on antimicrobial testing, including an example antibiogram.

In addition to antibiograms, the clinical microbiology laboratory is an essential partner in environmental testing. Although not routinely recommended due to cost, lack of standards, and possibility of inconclusive results, there may be situations in which testing is indicated, even required, including: biologic monitoring of sterilization processes, monthly cultures of water and dialysate in hemodialysis units, and short-term evaluation of the impact of infection measures or changes in infection prevention protocols.

When an epidemiologic investigation suggests that a source or reservoir of organisms may exist, special environmental testing may be needed. The decision to perform testing should be based on epidemiologic evidence indicating an association between the environment and host. Additionally, culturing for epidemiologic purposes should be systematic, specific, consistent, and part of a written infection prevention policy devised with input from the microbiology laboratory.

For outbreak situations, the clinical microbiology laboratory's role is vital and can perform important tasks providing further assistance to an investigation. These tasks include: confirming organism identities, identifying organism clusters, detecting new or unusual organisms and/or antimicrobial susceptibility patterns, retrieving archived microbiology data to determine background rates of organisms isolated, and determining the relatedness between isolates. These tasks can be completed through a variety of phenotypic and genotypic testing methods.

Lastly, the laboratory can help with the reporting of diseases (e.g., invasive *Streptococcus pneumoniae*). Most states have a public health code that requires certain infectious or communicable diseases and clinical syndromes be reported to the local state department of public health. Diseases are reportable based on their contagiousness, severity, or frequency. States set requirements for time and content of the reports.

The following table provides a general outline and examples of the additional, commonly utilized services/tests a clinical microbiology laboratory can provide. The table is broken down by the following:

- Laboratory test
- Indication for use
- Specific microbe
- Type of specimen
- Frequency (Note: The majority of this classification is as needed; however, there are exceptions.)
- Test type
- Interpretation of test
- Key points that include advantages and disadvantages of specific tests

Regardless of the test utilized, it is imperative for any infection prevention program to foster and build a collaborative relationship with the clinical microbiology laboratory in order to be successful in preventing HAIs and further development of antimicrobial resistance.

Table 11-1: Overview of Clinical Microbiology Lab Services and Tests

General Category	Laboratory Test	Indications	Specific Microbes	Specimen	Frequency	Test Type	Interpretation	Key Points
Antibiograms	Antimicrobial susceptibility testing (AST)	Recommended for all clinical microbiology laboratories, but required for clinical microbiology laboratory if accredited by College of American Pathologists (CAP)	All organisms, divided into Gram-negative and Gram-positive bacteria	Bacterial isolates	Annually	Minimal inhibitory concentration (MIC) breakpoint, defined for each bacterial species or genus by Clinical and Laboratory Standards Institute (CLSI), is the lowest concentration of a drug to which inhibits growth *in vitro*	Data organized into a summary table—total number of bacterial isolates tested against a range of antimicrobials and includes the percentage of bacterial isolates susceptible or resistant to each agent tested	• Advantages: Feasible, inexpensive; relatively rapid; able to track antimicrobial resistance levels and raise awareness, support use of optimal empiric therapy, and identify opportunities to reduce inappropriate antibiotic usage and to determine the effectiveness of those efforts • Disadvantages: Sometimes hospital population does not reflect community population, does not allow the susceptibility results to be evaluated by other potential variables (e.g., age, race, gender)
Environmental culturing	Culture of hospital water for *Legionellaceae*	• Generally not indicated except in cases of legionellosis or local regulation's requirement • Should be performed in accordance with published guidelines	*Legionella* spp.	Drinking water systems, cooling towers, evaporative condensers, hot water heaters, respiratory therapy equipment, etc.	As needed	Qualitative and quantitative culture using buffered charcoal yeast extract agar	• Presumptive identification: Colony characteristics, Gram stain reaction, and biotyping • Confirmatory identification: Immunofluorescence or slide agglutination	• Advantages: Can be compared to clinical isolates, detects all species and serogroups, 100% specific • Disadvantages: Technically difficult; slow to grow (>5 days); may not be performed in-house, but sent to a referral laboratory

Table 11-1: Overview of Clinical Microbiology Lab Services and Tests (continued)

General Category	Laboratory Test	Indications	Specific Microbes	Specimen	Frequency	Test Type	Interpretation	Key Points
	Culture and endotoxin assay of hemodialysis fluids	To validate the adequacy of the dialysis machine, disinfection process, and frequency	Identification is not required	• Minimum 50 mL • Dialysis water: Sample at point immediately past the water treatment system, where water exits storage tank, just before entry into dialysis machine, and water used to rinse dialyzers if applicable • Dialysate: From the effluent dialysate port on the dialyzer	• At least monthly • Repeat cultures when bacterial counts exceed the allowable level • Weekly for new systems or when changes are made	• Quantitative culture • Kinetic assay, gel clot assay, or single-tube test for endotoxin	• For quantitative culture: >50 colony-forming units (CFU)/mL, corrective action should be taken • For kinetic assay, gel clot assay or single-tube test for endotoxin: >1 endotoxin units (EU)/mL, corrective action should be taken	Disadvantages: Sensitivity highly dependent on technical skill
Environmental culturing *(continued)*	Air cultures for fungi	• Generally not indicated except in certain cases: when confirmed healthcare-associated infections (HAIs) due to environmental fungi occur, during construction, before initial occupancy of special controlled environments, or when procedures are in need of the cleanest air quality • Should be limited to environments with immunocompromised patients	Identification is not required if purpose is to determine presence/quantity, but if consideration is for source species, identification methods can be utilized	Air sampled by the following methods: sieve impactor, slit impactor, centrifugal impactor, impingers, filters, or settling plates	As needed	Quantitative culture using inhibitory mold agar with chloramphenicol (additional selective media may be used to differentiate fungi)	• Comparison of fungal levels between the controlled environmental areas and the uncontrolled areas or outdoors • Maximum allowed is <15 CFU/m³ for cultures incubated at room temperature and <2 CFU/m³ for 37°C	• Disadvantages: Technically difficult, sensitivity highly dependent on technical skill, slow to grow • Settling plates: Limited due to lack of quantification, most often sent to referral laboratory that specializes in this testing, most significant spores are too small and buoyant to settle
	Environmental and medical device surfaces	Generally not indicated except when determining effectiveness of new or modified cleaning/disinfecting products or in response to an epidemiologic investigation	Identification is not required if purpose is to determine presence/quantity, but if consideration is for source species, identification methods can be utilized	Samples obtained using the following methods: • Sample-rinse (swab, sponge, wipe) • Direct immersion • Containment (interior surfaces of containers, tubes, bottles, etc.) • Replicate organism detection and counting (RODAC) technique	As needed	Culture method	• Sample-rinse: report results by the area • Direct immersion: report results per item • Containment: evaluate both the type of organism and number of colonies • RODAC: quantitative; minimum of 15 plates per average hospital room	No standards available for interpretation, making testing questionable as to usefulness

Table 11-1: Overview of Clinical Microbiology Lab Services and Tests *(continued)*

General Category	Laboratory Test	Indications	Specific Microbes	Specimen	Frequency	Test Type	Interpretation	Key Points
Epidemiologic strain typing: Phenotypic	Biotyping	Presumptive identification	Variety of organisms	Bacterial isolates	As needed	The use of biochemical reactions, colony morphology, or nutritional and environmental requirements to differentiate organisms	Depends on type of test (e.g., oxidase producers)	Limited ability to determine relatedness between organisms
	AST	To determine an organism's susceptibility to certain antimicrobials	Variety of organisms	Bacterial isolates	As needed	MIC breakpoint, defined for each bacterial species or genus by CLSI: is the lowest concentration of a drug to which inhibits growth *in vitro*	Susceptible, intermediate, resistant, unknown	Relatively nonspecific and has limited ability to determine relatedness between organisms
Epidemiologic strain typing: Phenotypic *(continued)*	Serotyping	Determining relatedness of organisms	Variety of organisms	Bacterial isolates	As needed	Based on the antigenic components (outer membranes, flagella, capsules, etc.) of cell to differentiate	Agglutination	Requires purchase and storage of typing antisera, may not be readily available in most clinical microbiology laboratories
	Bacteriophage typing	Determining relatedness of organisms	Variety of organisms	Bacterial isolates	As needed	Identifies strains based on their patterns of susceptibility when introduced to a specific set of phages (viruses) that infect bacterial cells and cause lysis		• Most widely used with *Staphylococcus aureus* • Advantages: Range of utility • Disadvantages: Not easy to use and interpret, fair on reproducibility and discrimination, may not be readily available in most clinical microbiology laboratories

Table 11-1: Overview of Clinical Microbiology Lab Services and Tests *(continued)*

General Category	Laboratory Test	Indications	Specific Microbes	Specimen	Frequency	Test Type	Interpretation	Key Points
	Electrophoresis (e.g., polyacrylamide gel electrophoresis [PAGE], immunoblotting [Western blot], multilocus enzyme electrophoresis [MLEE])	Determining relatedness of organisms	Variety of organisms	Bacterial isolates	As needed	Detects differences in cellular proteins by molecular size by electrophoretically separating them in an acrylamide gel matrix resulting in a banding pattern	Bands are stained (rarely detected radioactively) and then compared (analyzed using mathematical algorithms in the case of MLEE)	• Advantages: Range of utility, reproducibility, ease of interpretation • Disadvantages: Labor intensive and time-consuming, may not be readily available in most clinical microbiology laboratories
Epidemiologic strain typing: Genotypic	Plasmid profile analysis (PPA)	Determining relatedness of organisms	Staphylococci, *Klebsiella, Enterobacter,* and *Serratia*	Bacterial isolates	As needed	Plasmids are collected from the organisms and restriction endonuclease digestion is performed, yielding enzyme-specific arrays of fragment sizes	Comparison of fragment sizes	• Advantages: Provides results in 1 day, allows for high-volume testing, variety of species can be analyzed, and is inexpensive • Disadvantages: Plasmids can be acquired or deleted, some organisms have no plasmids, may not be readily available in most clinical microbiology laboratories
Epidemiologic strain typing: Genotypic *(continued)*	Restriction endonuclease analysis (REA)	Determining relatedness of organisms	*Clostridium difficile*	Bacterial isolates	As needed	Restriction endonucleases are used to digest the entire chromosome resulting in enzyme-specific fragments	Comparison of fragments	May not be readily available in most clinical microbiology laboratories
	Southern blotting	Determining relatedness of organisms	Variety of organisms	Bacterial isolates	As needed	Restriction endonucleases are used to cut DNA strands, and then they are electrophoresed on agarose gel to separate by size	Comparison of fragments after treatment with radioactive, colorimetric, or chemiluminescently-labeled DNA probes	Disadvantages: Laborious and time-consuming, may not be readily available in most clinical microbiology laboratories

Table 11-1: Overview of Clinical Microbiology Lab Services and Tests *(continued)*

General Category	Laboratory Test	Indications	Specific Microbes	Specimen	Frequency	Test Type	Interpretation	Key Points
	Ribotyping	Determining relatedness of organisms	*Escherichia coli* and *S. aureus*	Bacterial isolates	As needed	Is a modification of the Southern blot-restriction fragment length polymorphism method using probes from the 16S and 23S rRNA genes of *E. coli*	Comparison of fragments	Disadvantages: Laborious and time-consuming, may not be readily available in most clinical microbiology laboratories
	Pulsed-field gel electrophoresis (PFGE)	Determining relatedness of organisms	Variety of organisms	Bacterial isolates	As needed	• Organisms embedded in agarose and lysed releasing chromosomal DNA, which is digested with restriction enzymes • Fragments are then separated by electrophoresis through the agarose matrix using a pulsed current, oriented diagonally, allowing for separation	Comparison of large genomic DNA fragments (DNA banding patterns)	• Advantages: Gold standard for molecular epidemiology, highly reproducible • Disadvantages: laborious, relative low through-put, requires precise standardization, and some organisms are highly clonal (identical) with only a limited number of patterns, therefore reducing the ability to differentiate, may not be readily available in most clinical microbiology laboratories

Table 11-1: Overview of Clinical Microbiology Lab Services and Tests *(continued)*

General Category	Laboratory Test	Indications	Specific Microbes	Specimen	Frequency	Test Type	Interpretation	Key Points
Epidemiologic strain typing: Genotypic *(continued)*	Amplification techniques (e.g., polymerase chain reaction [PCR]-based locus-specific restriction fragment length polymorphism [RFLP] typing, randomly amplified polymorphic DNA [RAPD] analysis, repetitive element [Rep]-PCR, cleavase fragment length polymorphism [CFLP], amplified fragment length polymorphism [AFLP], nucleic acid sequencing, multilocus sequence typing [MLST])	Determining relatedness of organisms	Variety of organisms	Bacterial isolates	As needed	Use of enzyme-mediated processes to synthesize copies of target nucleic acid	Depends on the test utilized (e.g., use of differential fluorescent labeling of nucleotides for nucleic acid sequencing)	• Advantages: Range of utility and reproducibility • Disadvantages Labor intensive and time-consuming, sensitive to contamination and false-positive reactions, may not be readily available in most clinical microbiology laboratories

References

Barnes S, Concepcion D, Felizardo G, et al. *Guide to the Elimination of Infections in Hemodialysis*. Washington, DC: Association for Professionals in Infection Control and Epidemiology, 2010.

Centers for Disease Control and Prevention. *Antibiogram Surveillance Method Using Cumulative Susceptibility Data*. Atlanta: CDC, 2005.

Hindler JF, Barton M, Callihan DR, et al. *Analysis and Presentation of Cumulative Antimicrobial Susceptibility Test Data: Approved Guideline*, 3rd ed. Wayne, PA: Clinical and Laboratory Standards Institute, 2009.

Courvalin P, LeClercq R, Rice LB, eds. *Antibiogram*. Washington, DC: American Society for Microbiology Press, 2009.

Gregson D, Church DE. Epidemiologic and Infection Control Microbiology. In: Garcia LS. *Clinical Microbiology Procedures Handbook*, 3rd ed. Washington, DC: American Society for Microbiology Press, 2010.

Murray PR. *Manual of Clinical Microbiology*, 10th ed. Washington, DC: American Society for Microbiology Press, 2011.

Moore V. Microbiology basics. In: Carrico R, et al., eds. *APIC Text of Infection Control and Epidemiology*, 3rd ed. Washington, DC: APIC, 2009:10–16.

Wenzel RP. *Prevention and Control of Nosocomial Infections*, 4th ed. Philadelphia: Lippincott Williams & Wilkins, 2003.

Glossary of Abbreviations

AFB	Acid-fast bacillus (bacilli)
AFLP	Amplified fragment length polymorphism
AMI	Acute myocardial infarction
ANC	Absolute neutrophil count
ANSI	American National Standards Institute
AST	Antimicrobial Susceptibility Testing
APTT	Activated partial thromboplastin time
BAL	Bronchoalveolar lavage
BCYE	Buffered charcoal yeast extract
BUN	Blood urea nitrogen
CAP	College of American Pathologists
CFLP	Cleavase fragment length polymorphism
CFU	Colony-forming unit
CHF	Congestive heart failure
CK	Creatine kinase
CLIA	Clinical Laboratory Improvement Amendments
CLSI	Clinical and Laboratory Standards Institute
CMV	Cytomegalovirus
COPD	Chronic obstructive pulmonary disease
CSF	Cerebrospinal fluid
DFA	Direct fluorescent antibody
DIC	Disseminated intravascular coagulation
DML	Diagnostic microbiology laboratory
EBV	Epstein-Barr virus
EEE/ EEV	Eastern equine encephalitis or equine encephalitis virus
EIA	Enzyme immunoassay
ESBL	Extended-spectrum beta-lactamase
ESR	Erythrocyte sedimentation rate
FDA	Food and Drug Administration
GBS	Group B streptococcus
GGT	Gamma-glutamyl transferase
GI	Gastrointestinal
GLC	Gas liquid chromatography
HAI	Healthcare-associated infection
HBV	Hepatitis B virus
HCV	Hepatitis C virus
HHV-6	Human herpes virus 6
HIV	Human immunodeficiency virus
HPLC	High pressure liquid chromatography
HPV	Human papilloma virus
HSV	Herpes simplex virus

IgG	Immunoglobulin
IP	Infection Preventionist
JCV	John Cunningham virus
KPC	Klebsiella pneumoniae carbapenemase
LDH	Lactate dehydrogenase
LRI	Lower respiratory infection
MCH	Mean corpuscular hemoglobin
MCHC	Mean corpuscular hemoglobin concentration
MDRO	Multidrug-resistant organisms
MI	Myocardial infarction
MIC	Minimal inhibitory concentration
MIRU-VNTR	Mycobacterial interspersed repetitive units - Variable number of tandem repeats
MLEE	Multilocus enzyme electrophoresis
MLST	Multilocus sequence typing
MOTT	Mycobacteria other than tuberculosis
MOV	Mean platelet volume
MRSA	Methicillin-resistant Staphylococcus aureaus
MTB	Mycobacteria tuberculosis
NAA	Nucleic acid amplification
NDM-1	New Delhi metallo-beta-lactamase
NP	Nasopharyngeal
PAGE	Polyacrylamide gel electrophoresis
PAS	Periodic acid-Schiff
PCR	Polymerase chain reaction
PFGE	Pulsed-field gel electrophoresis
PMN	Polymorphonuclear neutrophils
POC	Point of care
PPA	Plasmid profile analysis
PPE	Personal protective equipment
PT	Prothrombin time
PTT	Partial thromboplastin time
RAPD	Randomly amplified polymorphic DNA
RDW	Red blood cell distribution width
REA	Restriction endonuclease analysis
RFLP	Restriction fragment length polymorphism
RSV	Respiratory syncytial virus
RT	Room temperature
SARS-CoV	Severe acute respiratory syndrome coronavirus
SG	Specific gravity
SLE	St. Louis encephalitis
SSI	Surgical site infection
TCT	Thrombin clotting time
TRH	Thyrotropin-releasing hormone
TSH	Thyroid-stimulating hormone
TT	Thrombin time
UA	Urinalysis

UTI	Urinary tract infection
VZV	Vericella zoster virus
WBC	White blood cell
WNV	West Nile virus